TAKING
CHARGE

TAKING
CHARGE

*Overcoming the Challenges
of Long-Term Illness*

IRENE POLLIN, M.S.W.,
with
Susan K. Golant, M.A.

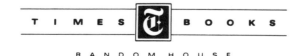

TIMES 𝕿 BOOKS

RANDOM HOUSE

To my daughter, Linda Joy,
who woke with a smile
every morning of her life

Library of Congress Cataloging-in-Publication Data

Pollin, Irene
    Taking charge : overcoming the challenges of long-term illness Irene Pollin, with Susan K. Golant.—1st ed.
        p.   cm.
    Includes bibliographical references and index.
    ISBN 0-8129-2258-1
    1. Chronic diseases—Psychological aspects.   I. Golant, Susan K. II. Title.
    RC108.P65   1994
    616'.001'9—dc20

                                                            93-29434

Text design by Levavi & Levavi
Manufactured in the United States of America

9 8 7 6 5 4 3 2

First Edition

THE THIRD PACIFIC TRADE
AND DEVELOPMENT CONFERENCE
SYDNEY 1970

DIRECT FOREIGN INVESTMENT
IN ASIA AND THE PACIFIC

Acknowledgments

I had considered writing this book for many years, but the final impetus to begin came from two dear friends who are themselves writers. Their display of confidence in my ability to write what I knew and felt so passionately about was the catalyst. Sue Tolchin and Ruth Boorstin, both members of my wonderful book club, offered me sound advice and listened to my complaints. Another member of the same club, Jessica Josephson, referred me to my agent, Nick Ellison. Jessica also pumped me up whenever I felt deflated—and that was often. Nick Ellison turned out to be the best thing that ever happened to me because he never failed me. There were a number of quite difficult moments and I appreciate his unfailing loyalty, support, and perseverance. Without him, this book would never have been published.

Sue Golant, my co-author, also came along at a time when I had just about burned out. She revived both me and the book. She had the energy that I had used up. This book would not have been completed without her. She was absolutely the right person for me to work with, and I wish to thank her here.

I am indebted to a small number of colleagues who read early manuscripts carefully and gave me exceedingly valuable criticism when I needed it: Dr. Fawzy Fawzy of UCLA, Dr. James Strain of Mount Sinai Hospital of New York, Dr. Ruth McCorkle of the University of Pennsylvania, Dr. Marguerite Lederberg and Dr. Jimmie Holland of Memorial Sloan-Kettering Hospital, and Dr. Michael Jellinek of Massachusetts General Hospital.

I am grateful to the patients with whom I have worked over the years. Many of their stories appear here, although I have changed their names and identifying characteristics to protect their privacy.

I am also grateful to two people who are the closest to me: my friend Cherry Adler, who never let me give up, and my dearest husband, Abe Pollin, who lived with my ups and downs and dried my tears. He always understood my need to complete this project.

Ultimately, I was exceptionally fortunate in having Betsy Rapoport as my editor. She was absolutely the right person for me and the book. And I would also like to acknowledge Peter Osnos, my publisher, for his vision and energy.

Finally, the inspiration for this book was the life and death at age sixteen of my daughter, Linda Joy. Born with a severe heart defect, she had a love of life and living and awoke each morning with a smile on her face. I never heard her complain that life was unfair. Life was what it was for her. She had to face the possibility of death when she agreed to open heart surgery, and she never flinched. She was a magnificent human being with much love and wisdom to give but not enough time to do it. I still miss her very much.

IRENE POLLIN, M.S.W.
Chevy Chase, Maryland

For my part, I am deeply grateful for having had the opportunity to work with Irene Pollin. Her sensitivity, generosity of spirit, commitment to the ideas expressed in this book, and resourcefulness in carrying them out have served as a model to me. She has touched many lives (including mine) with her warmth and kindness and by dint of *Taking Charge*, will touch many, many more.

I would also like to thank members of Irene Pollin's staff: Sharon Hildebrandt, Executive Director of the Linda Pollin Foundation, and Cleo Neiman, Ms. Pollin's assistant. They have been most helpful in sending me research and materials and have responded to my (sometimes frantic) requests graciously and professionally. Susan Baird Kanaan, M.S.W., my counterpart in the writing of a book for professionals, has been a wonderful sounding board and ally.

As always, I am grateful to my agent, Bob Tabian, for watching over my interests. I would also like to thank our editor, Betsy Rapoport, for her unstinting support and praise of our efforts.

Finally, I am grateful to my family. My husband, Dr. Mitch Golant, as vice president of program at the Wellness Community, National, has taught me much about the needs of cancer patients and their families. But more than that, he is and always has been my dearest friend and most ardent supporter. Without him, my writing career would have been impossible.

And I am also grateful to my parents, Arthur and Mary Kleinhandler. Survivors of Buchenwald and Dachau, they have always managed, with humor, intelligence, and great tenacity, to overcome whatever difficulties—medical or otherwise—have been thrown in their path. They have inspired me with their love, their deep appreciation of the miracle of life, and their ability to make the best of things and go on, despite it all.

For these and other gifts I am grateful.

SUSAN K. GOLANT, M.A.
West Los Angeles, California

of spirit, commitment to the ideas expressed in this book, and resourcefulness in carrying them out have served as a model to me. She has touched many lives (including mine) with her warmth and kindness and by dint of *Taking Charge*, will touch many, many more.

I would also like to thank members of Irene Pollin's staff: Sharon Hildebrandt, Executive Director of the Linda Pollin Foundation, and Cleo Neiman, Ms. Pollin's assistant. They have been most helpful in sending me research and materials and have responded to my (sometimes frantic) requests graciously and professionally. Susan Baird Kanaan, M.S.W., my counterpart in the writing of a book for professionals, has been a wonderful sounding board and ally.

As always, I am grateful to my agent, Bob Tabian, for watching over my interests. I would also like to thank our editor, Betsy Rapoport, for her unstinting support and praise of our efforts.

Finally, I am grateful to my family. My husband, Dr. Mitch Golant, as vice president of program at the Wellness Community, National, has taught me much about the needs of cancer patients and their families. But more than that, he is and always has been my dearest friend and most ardent supporter. Without him, my writing career would have been impossible.

And I am also grateful to my parents, Arthur and Mary Kleinhandler. Survivors of Buchenwald and Dachau, they have always managed, with humor, intelligence, and great tenacity, to overcome whatever difficulties—medical or otherwise—have been thrown in their path. They have inspired me with their love, their deep appreciation of the miracle of life, and their ability to make the best of things and go on, despite it all.

For these and other gifts I am grateful.

SUSAN K. GOLANT, M.A.
West Los Angeles, California

Contents

Contents

Part I

YOUR NEW
REALITY

1.

Confronting Your Medical Crisis

If you are suffering from a long-term illness, it may be of some comfort to recognize that *you are not alone.* You may not know that:

- As of 1993, the Arthritis Foundation estimates that 37 million Americans are living with the disease; that's one of every seven people. Arthritis strikes one in three U.S. families.
- The American Diabetes Association estimates that as of 1992, 14 million Americans are coping with diabetes.
- According to the American Heart Association, more than 6 million Americans alive today have a history of heart disease. In addition, nearly a million individuals have been coping with congenital heart defects.
- The U.S. Department of Health and Human Services documents more than a million new cases of cancer *each year.*

- The National Multiple Sclerosis Society estimates that well over a quarter of a million Americans live with multiple sclerosis (MS).
- In 1989 (the most recent year for which statistics are available), 190,000 people were treated for kidney failure.

Although we all recognize examples of long-term or chronic illness such as arthritis and diabetes, the term *chronic illness* itself is not easily defined. Not too long ago, for example, cancer was thought of as an acute and fatal condition; yet today this disease is also considered a chronic illness, since many cancer patients survive for years with their malady. In fact, a chronic illness can be incapacitating or not; gradual or sudden in onset; fatal, potentially life-shortening, or inconsequential to one's life span; progressive or unchanging.

Some incapacitating diseases such as diabetes, kidney disease, and Graves' disease can be controlled with medication and other treatments.

The National Center for Health Statistics considers a condition chronic if it lasts more than three months. A chronic "impairment" is usually permanent and can result from a disease, injury, or congenital condition.

The good news is that today many of us live longer and more productive lives than our grandparents and great-grandparents ever dreamed possible. Nevertheless, because of our lengthening life spans, we run a greater risk of con-tracting long-term ailments, many of which can be con-trolled by ongoing medical attention. As our population ages, it is likely that more and more of us will be living with long-term conditions of one sort or another. It is a virtual certainty that you or someone you know will be affected by long-term illness.

Because some illnesses can continue for years, you and your family may find yourselves dealing with not only the medical side of the disease but also its social and emotional impact on your lives. While physicians generally focus on their patients' physical condition, the psychological consequences can be devastating as well.

Research suggests that individuals with long-term illnesses have a greater incidence of emotional distress than those who are well. If you are ill, for example, you may become fearful and depressed or enraged. You may withdraw from friends and family—the support network you so sorely need at this vulnerable time—out of a fear of dependency, abandonment, or stigmatization. You may even perceive your health as being worse than it actually is; when you first receive your diagnosis, you may be unaware of its implications, the available treatments, or your innate coping skills.

How to cope effectively with your long-term illness is the subject of this book. I have written it to offer guidance and support in overcoming the fears and emotional hurdles that may interfere with your leading a full and rewarding life, despite your disease. *Coping is a process that occurs over time and not overnight.* In reading *Taking Charge*, your goal should be not to cure your illness (for that may be impossible), but rather to learn how to live with it.

WHO AM I?

A licensed psychiatric social worker based in Washington, D.C., I have specialized in counseling individuals with long-term diseases and their families since 1974. I come by my deep belief in the necessity of such support from personal experience. In 1952, my son Kenneth Jay died at the age of thirteen months of a congenital heart ailment. Even more tragically, in 1963, my daughter, Linda, died at the age of sixteen. Linda's death, though a terrible shock, was not entirely a surprise, for Linda had suffered from a steadily worsening congenital heart problem similar to the one Kenneth had had. She did not survive a second, then experimental, open heart surgery to save and prolong her life.

As you can imagine, the loss of one child was extraordinarily painful. The loss of two, almost unimaginable. I sought counseling after my daughter died and saw several well-trained professionals. Some prescribed tranquilizers, which served only to mask my feelings, not resolve them. Other therapists, rather than recognizing my children's illnesses and deaths as the source of my unhappiness, questioned me about my childhood. This approach annoyed me. I had had a very fine childhood, thank you very much! What did that have to do with what I was struggling with now?

What I needed (and wasn't getting) from these counselors was help in coping with the long-term effects of heart disease on me and on my family. It was then that I realized that mental health professionals receive little training specifically designed for those dealing with chronic illnesses. Few therapists are attuned to their *special needs.*

Indeed, as a result of my personal experience, I now champion the belief that the chronically ill deserve more emotional support than they are receiving from the medical establishment. Nine years after my daughter's death, I returned to school to complete a master's degree in psychiatric social work. And then I began to develop a special kind of counseling tailored specifically to the needs of the chronically ill. I named it "medical crisis counseling" because I wanted the focus to be on the *medical crisis,* not on personal or family history. During medical crisis counseling, I help my patients explore how their illness has affected their lives as well as those of their families. The medical crisis is the catalyst for their seeking help. The counseling is focused and short-term, as little as one session and usually no more than twelve, although patients can return from time to time, as needed.

In order to further this concept, I became the founder and director of the Department of Social Services at the Neurology Center, a large private neurology practice in Chevy Chase, Maryland, and subsequently the founder and for three years executive director of the Outpatient Medical Crisis Counseling Center at Washington Hospital Center, a large inner-city hospital in Washington, D.C. In addition to a private practice devoted to the emotional care of the chronically ill, I have supervised other counselors and given workshops on the social and emotional needs of the chronically ill to community health agencies, professional organizations, and academic institutions.

I also founded and am the president of the Linda Pollin Foundation which, with Children's Hospital in Boston (affiliated with Harvard University), supports the training of mental health professionals in their attention to the social and emotional needs of chronically ill patients. The Linda Pollin Foundation, in conjunction with the National Institute of Mental Health, conducts yearly conferences with physicians, psychiatrists, psychologists, and other health professionals around the country to implement and support medical crisis counseling in hospital and private practice settings nationwide. A presidential appointee to the National Cancer Institute, I was also chair of its Subcommittee on Women's Health.

From my life experience, research, clinical practice, and involvement with the medical establishment and federal health institutes, I have discovered that by confronting and taking charge of your fears, you can learn to accept your long-term condition. Indeed, you can once again take charge of your life. This book will show you the way.

YOUR MEDICAL CRISIS

If you have been diagnosed recently with a long-term illness, you and your loved ones will most likely experience (perhaps for the first time in your lives) a wide range of powerful and painful emotions such as anxiety, terror, denial, anger, depression, helplessness, frustration, and even shame. These feelings are *normal and expectable* in your situation. They are a *natural* response to a personal catastrophe of such enormous proportions. (It would be entirely unnatural, for example, for you to feel relaxed or happy upon being told that your mystifying symptoms stem from multiple sclerosis!) These feelings can signal an emotional reaction to a medical crisis.

These crises occur most often in three situations:

1. *The diagnosis of a long-term condition.* Sitting in the doctor's office as she breaks the news, you may find yourself in a state of shock, as if in the midst of a nightmare from which you cannot awaken. You believe your world has collapsed. You may stop listening as the knowledge that your life has been changed forever resonates throughout your being. Indeed, research has shown that people who have just been diagnosed with a serious illness such as melanoma may feel just as stressed, if not more so, as patients who face a bone marrow transplant—a treatment of last resort. Often, we let our imaginations run wild and visualize the worst possible outcome immediately after diagnosis.

2. *Flare-ups.* You may have accepted your illness and adjusted to it in its present manifestation when suddenly, and perhaps inexplicably, it worsens. Again, you may feel thrown into a maelstrom of difficult and painful emotions from which you see no escape.

3. *Soon after release from the hospital.* Safe and secure when cared for by professional and practiced hands, you may lack expert support once you are home. Loved ones may be unable to cope. You may feel physically weak or frightened. The trauma of surgery may heighten your vulnerability and awareness of mortality.

Moreover, individuals with differing diseases experience their medical crises differently. An epileptic may fear, for example, social stigmatization at the loss of consciousness and uncontrollable behavior resulting from a seizure in public. Patients with serious respiratory ailments such as cystic fibrosis may feel reluctant to sleep because they fear suffocating in the middle of the night. Those whose kidneys have failed may fear that the hemodialysis machine upon which they depend will assume control of their lives or will break down in the middle of a treatment. Those who have been diagnosed with cancer simply fear that they will die a slow and agonizing death. All of these fears are normal and valid and all can and should be dealt with.

ADDRESSING YOUR FEARS

Despite the overwhelming nature of your illness and its psychological consequences to you and your family, there is hope. Research has found that anger and hostility raise blood pressure and weaken the immune system. But psychological counseling tailored to the needs of the chronically ill can be beneficial for your mental and physical health. In the case of heart disease, for example, counseling can reduce the recurrence of heart attacks, high blood pressure, the length of your hospital stay, anxiety, and complications. Counseling is designed to lessen tension, which slows down the heart rate. Any activity that reduces stress, particularly in the long term, increases a sense of well-being.

The positive contributions of counseling for people with cancer is equally dramatic. In fact, researchers have found that cancer patients in group support situations experience less emotional distress, depression, anxiety, failure to cope, tension, fatigue, anger, and confusion than those who are not involved in support groups.

One team of doctors led by David Spiegel, M.D., at Stanford University, discovered that women with metastatic breast cancer (breast cancer that has spread to other organs in the body) who had participated in a cancer support group lived twice as long as those who just received medical care without the psychosocial counseling. The researchers concluded that the emotional support reduced stress by breaking the cycle of social alienation that so often occurs with cancer patients. Improved diet, careful compliance with doctors' orders, and a strengthened immune system may all emanate from this kind of support.

But what if counseling is unavailable in your area? Or what if you find, as I did, that the mental health professionals you've consulted simply don't have the training to help you, never having been confronted by an epilepsy or kidney patient before? Or what if you shy away from any form of psychotherapy, fearing you'd be stigmatized as "crazy" or "weak" if you seek relief for your current emotional distress? Finally, what if, in your time of difficulty, you simply cannot afford the additional financial strain of ongoing therapy?

While these are stumbling blocks, they certainly are not insurmountable. I've written this book so that you can take advantage of my experience and understanding, even if counseling is otherwise unavailable or if you're reluctant to go to someone's office to receive it. It is my hope that you will use *Taking Charge* as a means of coping with the feelings that your chronic illness have evoked.

THE EIGHT FEARS
OF CHRONIC ILLNESSES

As a result of my working with hundreds of patients and scores of mental health professionals, I have come to see that most people in your position must grapple at one time or another with eight distinct fears.

In Part II of *Taking Charge*, I will examine each of these fears in depth. For the moment, however, let's preview them so that you understand the phases of your emotional reactions as they are likely to develop. Bear in mind that while these eight fears develop in roughly the same sequence for most people, as a unique individual, you may experience them in a somewhat altered order or you may experience several at once. And because of your own personality and life experience, you may find some fears easier to confront than others.

From my experience, the eight fears of chronic illnesses are:

1. The fear of loss of control. If you are facing a long-term illness, you may feel that you are standing on ever shifting ground; feelings of being in control and helplessness change places frequently. Indeed, people who are chronically ill and their families often seek out professional help because they feel overwhelmed by the fear that they have lost control over their lives due to the disease. They wish to regain what has been lost. *Taking Charge* will teach you and your family how to reassert control over your lives the next time you feel overwhelmed.

2. The fear of loss of self-image. If you are coping with a long-term illness, you must face the fact that you no longer view yourself as the same person. The new image isn't necessarily worse, but it is different. At first, you may feel less confident or less attractive, physically weaker or somehow damaged. These feelings can and will change. Indeed, your image of yourself will evolve as your emphasis shifts from external to internal traits. Your looks or physical prowess may now take second place to improved personal relationships. As you confront who you really are, you may discover your value not in superficial criteria but in your true self.

Once you confront these issues by having realistic expectations of yourself, you will become comfortable with your different self.

3. *The fear of dependency.* The fear of dependency usually manifests itself once the reality of the illness sinks in and we recognize that our condition is not going to disappear. Most of us fear becoming dependent on another, especially in a society that values the "rugged individual"—the lone cowboy who makes his way across the Old West or the widow who raises her eight children single-handedly. Hating to show any vulnerability, we may have difficulty accepting that we will need or have to ask for outside help. Conversely, we may also fear being depended upon. Again, once we confront and accept this potent fear, we can begin to address our dependency needs. Indeed, *Taking Charge* will teach you about a positive kind of dependency: an interdependency that is based on mutual needs.

4. *The fear of stigma.* You may become apprehensive that others in your world will disparage you or distance themselves from you once they know that you are sick, as if illness brings with it some sort of shame. In other instances, you may fear that others will point and stare, especially if your illness causes some outwardly apparent physical disabilities. The fear of stigma differs from that of a changed self-image because stigma arises from the way society views you, rather than the way you view yourself. Stigma is external while self-image is internal. In *Taking*

Charge, you will learn how to plan for and confront the fear of stigma and the stigma itself realistically.

5. *The fear of abandonment.* This is a primitive fear that many of us carry from our childhoods. As infants, we were apprehensive that our parents wouldn't be available or loving when we needed them. Once we are ill, however, the fear of abandonment takes on new dimensions. Even in the most affectionate and giving of families, we may grow frightened that our spouse, siblings, children, or other loved ones will tire of the drudgery that our care entails. This normal and universal anxiety stems from the disease having threatened our personal sense of security.

I have found, however, that once this worry is understood, most come to recognize it as only a fear and nothing more. Indeed, you may even learn that, contrary to your worst fears, your loved ones find caregiving the source of a great deal of personal satisfaction. It may give them a sense of control and accomplishment in an uncontrollable situation. Or they may feel that they're doing everything they can to assuage their own anxiety and perhaps some repressed guilt.

6. *The fear of expressing anger.* When you realize that you have done everything possible yet you can never cure your disease, you may become intensely angry. In *Anger: The Misunderstood Emotion,* social psychologist Carol Tavris explains that anger is a response to frustration. In the case of a long-term illness, it's evident why such a definition would easily apply: anger is a normal and expectable reaction to long-term illness. Yet many people shrink from expressing the anger they must surely feel because they've been taught that anger is an unwelcome emotion. Or they may suppress their rage for fear of flying out of control. Such stifled anger can cause depression and sap energy.

Taking Charge provides strategies to help you accept and express your anger appropriately, without doing damage to yourself or your loved ones.

7. *The fear of isolation.* Physical, social, and emotional isolation can result from a long-term illness. If you are physically confined, you may lack the ability to socialize with old friends and may find yourself withdrawing further from them. The fear of isolation often occurs after you have been ill for a while, usually because it takes time to pull away from society or to recognize that your friends, family, acquaintances, and coworkers are avoiding you. Yet, as you will see, medical crisis counseling offers personal solutions, such as airing your feelings in order to maintain old relationships or joining a peer support group.

8. *The fear of death.* Although people who are diagnosed with a serious long-term illness fear death, ironically, it is not what they fear the most. Rather, our greatest fears revolve around how we will live with our chronic illness until we die, be it a matter of months or even decades. Once you recognize that your fear of dying is in truth a fear of living, you will confront the real issue and shift your focus to solving the problems of everyday life.

Once you have gone through these eight fears, you should discover that they are less frightening. You have anticipated and faced the worst.

THE GOALS OF THIS BOOK

Medical crisis counseling is designed to help you to understand why you're feeling the way you do and to realize that your emotions are normal, natural, and predictable. It is also meant to encourage you to get back on your feet again. I will assist you in redefining your self-concept in the context of your new situation and renewing your zest for living within the unexplored definition of yourself. You will be adjusting your behavior and attitude rather than your personality.

As a chronically ill person, you must ultimately come to terms with the reality of your situation. You must discard false hopes and restructure your life based on your present capabilities and limitations. To that end, in the course of reading *Taking Charge,* I will help you and your family to:

- Identify your coping style.
- Gain a perspective on your problems and accept your stress and emotional reaction as normal.
- Set realistic and reachable goals that will put you back in charge of your life.
- Identify your own strengths and weaknesses, likes and dislikes, beliefs and values, and "shoulds" and "should nots," as well as which relationships and activities you can maintain despite your illness.
- Maximize your personal and environmental resources: physical strength, psychological stamina, support networks, and knowledge.
- Adapt to your illness.
- Decrease your anxiety and distress.
- Maintain and improve your daily functioning.
- Improve your cooperation with your doctors and nurses by understanding the framework from which they operate.
- Reduce isolation and withdrawal from one another, your community, and your work.
- Regain a sense of control.
- Improve your satisfaction and the quality of your life.

Although these goals are lofty, they have been achieved by many of my patients and can be achieved with your thoughtful hard work.

HOW TO USE THIS BOOK

As a therapist, I understand that reading a book is no substitute for your meeting with a live person in a counseling session regularly. I cannot make the eye contact or read other body language that signal understanding, emotional support, or confusion. It's difficult for me to give advice and make sure that you understand my points without seeing your face and hearing your questions. Because such dialogue is impossible in a book, I have sought to anticipate your concerns and fears, questions and triumphs.

But since you are getting counseling advice from a book, I am going to ask you to do a few things as you read. First, just pretend you're sitting in my office. It's a pleasant and inviting place. Imagine that you're in a chair facing me and that you're telling me how you feel and what you're afraid of. I am in a chair with my feet on a small stool, facing you. I am giving you my complete attention, listening carefully to your every word. It should feel good because I am a trained listener.

If you think of questions you'd like to ask me or concerns you'd like to air, write them down on a sheet of paper, in a journal, or in the margins of this book. Put asterisks next to the issues you'd like to comment upon or think about further. If what I write upsets you or if you disagree with it, write these points down too and then move on. Don't dwell on them. If you return to these issues later, you may find they hold a different meaning for you.

You can also use your notes in the margins to communicate your thoughts to a family member or friend with whom you have been unable to articulate your deepest feelings. You may, in this indirect way, spark a new and perhaps more healing dialogue.

Throughout *Taking Charge*, I have written about some of the people whom I was able to help, what I did with them

and why. I also tell of my own struggles, some quite difficult, especially since I didn't have a trained counselor to
help me. Reading about the dilemmas others have faced
helps you become more aware of your own feelings.

I want you to be aware of the struggles that my patients
and I experienced. So many self-help books paint such a
rosy picture of success that while you're reading them you
may feel you can't match the author's performance. You
may even try and then find, much to your consternation,
that the suggested program doesn't work for you. This may
leave you feeling inadequate or even like a failure.

As you read, I want you to realize that the struggle you
are facing is difficult and painful. Coping with a long-term
illness may become easier over time but it never disappears
entirely. Better to be prepared for the long haul than to have
unrealistic expectations and dashed hopes. During the
struggle, it helps to recognize that you are coping even
when you think you aren't! For example, you may consider
crying all day as "not coping" but crying may be just what
you need to do. Coping is dynamic—it's an ongoing process
and you're in the midst of it. It's only when you judge the
process as being bad that you undermine your own
progress.

Taking Charge follows the usual progression of emotions
when one is diagnosed with a long-term illness. Part I helps
you examine your coping style, how it feels when you first
discover the disease, your family's response, and your experience in dealing with physicians. In Part II, I will help you
to confront and resolve each of the eight fears of long-term
illness. You need not read *Taking Charge* in one sitting or
straight through, chapter by chapter. You may feel more
comfortable reading selectively about the fears that trouble
you or the issues that interest you the most. Some concerns
may overlap in your mind and some may be more promi-
nent than others. This is natural. And don't expect to solve

all of your problems at once. This may be too overwhelming. Choose one at a time.

My single most important piece of advice: Give yourself enough time to consider what I've written and especially your own responses, good and bad. If the book upsets you, set it aside for a while. If you find an insight valuable, savor it. If you come to a better understanding of your situation and your options, then I will have accomplished what I have set out to do.

2.

Coping with Your Long-Term Illness

Coping with a long-term illness is essentially different from anything you may have encountered before. With an acute disease such as influenza, appendicitis, or gallstones you can plan for a time when your life will return to normal. "How long will it take?" is a question your doctor can answer with some certitude. Within a definable period of time you will be cured. You will likely never have to deal with this affliction again.

With long-term illness, however, there is no cure in the traditional sense, only remission. Medication and surgery can extend and improve the quality of your life, but the state of "normalcy" you once knew may never return. Moreover, your disease could recur someday, necessitating your dealing with it again. In the past, there were solutions, now only adjustment and acceptance. Rather than being certain, the future becomes clouded and unknown; it seems frightening.

Although your life has been altered permanently, you can find the strength and courage to go on. Think of the amputees, epileptics, or diabetics who participate in marathons or ski competitions. These people have integrated their illness—*it no longer dominates their lives.* Although difficult, integration is possible.

All people struggling with long-term illnesses face essentially the same set of problems and fears but their coping styles are individual; there are as many ways of coping as there are people in the world. In order to adjust to your illness, it may help to go through the following seven-step process. Think of it as a road map of possible coping strategies:

1. Identify your problems.
2. Take stock.
3. Face your fears.
4. Find a way to release tension.
5. Acknowledge and work within your own coping style.
6. Understand that adjustment occurs in an ebb and flow.
7. Recognize and appreciate integration when it occurs.

Let's examine these steps more closely to help you in your adjustment process.

IDENTIFY YOUR PROBLEMS

Knowledge is power. In order to handle the problems you're bound to encounter, you must first be aware of them. As painful as it may be, with awareness comes the possibility of adjustment, integration, and resolution. Without it, you may become stuck, confused, or embittered. With insight, however, you can anticipate the rough spots. Because you can expect certain challenges, you prepare for them and learn how to handle them, thus diminishing their effect on you.

To help visualize the complexity of problems inherent in coping with long-term illnesses, picture a pane of safety glass that has been hit very hard by a sharp object such as a small stone. The glass doesn't shatter and fall to the ground. Instead, immediately around the center of impact, a web of fine cracks appears. The network grows, radiating in every direction. Some fissures are short, others long. Some spread directly from the center while others intersect. All the fractures are connected, even those at the farthest edges of the pane, because they result from the same impact. Although the glass is more fragile than before it was hit, it still remains whole in its fractured state.

So it is with your long-term illness. You will encounter a myriad of intersecting medical, social, emotional, and economic problems. There are the obvious physical disabilities to overcome: pain; restricted movement, activities, or diet; dependency on medication and medical technology, to name a few. In addition, your relationship with family and friends may change. You'll confront the often intimidating medical profession. Your income and savings may diminish, possibly altering your social status. Your loved ones—the major source of emotional support—may feel as vulnerable and helpless as you.

Anyone who denies being overwhelmed at this time is simply not telling the truth. Yet even as you consider the number of problems resulting from the impact of long-term illness on your life, you'll recognize that although weakened and perhaps impaired, you remain the same person. Like the pane of glass, you've been hard hit but you are whole and you are capable of adjusting to the fate you have been dealt.

Consider making a flow chart or diagram showing (and concretizing) the intersection of the problems arising from your illness as the fissures in a cracked pane of glass. Put your illness in the middle and draw and label the issues you must deal with as lines radiating from the center or intersecting with one another. Then draw a circle around your design to show that wholeness still exists, despite the disease. This exercise can help you bring your own problems into focus, so you'll know what you're up against.

TAKE STOCK

You may also find it useful to take a personal history of your illness, much the way a therapist might do. This will help you assess your weaknesses as well as your strengths.

Answer the following questions in a journal or on a sheet of paper:

1. What is your disease, its stage and prognosis at this time?
2. What was your reaction to the original diagnosis? How long ago was that? How do you feel about it now?
3. How were you and your family feeling emotionally before the diagnosis? How did you feel after it?
4. How much of your "normal" life can you carry on despite your illness? What modifications have you had to make in daily social, work, or family routines?
5. What would you say are your physical strengths and weaknesses today? Are they any different than before you became ill?
6. Who can you turn to for support in times of need: family, friends, community, social service agencies, self-help groups?
7. Are there other major stressors occurring in your home separate from your illness, such as a child going off to college, job loss, moving, or the illness or recent death of an elderly parent?

Once you have made this assessment, you can call on this information as you read this book. I will be bringing up related issues along the way.

FACE YOUR FEARS

Many people worry that if they confront their fears, they'll fall apart or lose control. In truth, all of us wish to be secure in what we know we can count on. It feels safe and reassuring to have a sense of control. However, it doesn't follow automatically that if you're frightened or unsure of what's in store you'll be out of control.

Every day, uncertainty slips into our lives. Neither a salesperson nor a department store buyer knows in advance how many items they'll sell, yet they order merchandise. A restaurateur shops for and prepares meals by predicting how many patrons will order roast beef or fish or lasagne in a given evening—but he never knows for sure. There is an expectation of certainty, but in fact no one is certain the expectation will be fulfilled.

While we can conduct business tolerating a measure of ambiguity, we find it hard to apply these principles to our health. We want to be sure we're healthy yet we can never really be completely confident. What goes on within our bodies is often invisible to us. We don't recognize a problem until it becomes a bleeding ulcer or shortness of breath. In truth, we live with uncertainty all the time, yet we maintain control of our lives.

Nevertheless, "fear of falling apart" pushes people to keep their other anxieties inside, even when it means going against their natural tendency to face them and express themselves openly. For example, Emily, one of my young patients from Chicago, became uncharacteristically silent after a diagnosis of multiple sclerosis. Her husband felt so uncomfortable with her atypical demeanor that he finally screamed at her, "For God's sake, Emily, you've got MS. Where's your reaction?"

All her life, Emily had prided herself on her ability to communicate. Now, however, she feared losing control if she verbalized her terrifying thoughts: "Will I end up in a wheelchair?" "Will I be able to have children?" "If I do have kids, will they have to care for me or make the decision to put me in a nursing home?" Once she allowed herself to voice these terrible but understandable fears to herself and her husband, not only did she feel more stable emotionally, but she was able to make decisions about her life that eased her adjustment to her new situation.

In Part II, I'll be helping you face and resolve your fears by examining the most salient ones in detail. One of the fears I don't cover—what I like to call the "ninth fear"—asserts that you're making up all the others. This attitude can undermine your ability to accept your other anxieties as legitimate. When you succumb to it, you don't permit yourself to be serious about or respectful of your own needs.

Let me assure you that even though in the past some of your fears may have been unfounded, today they are valid. They're based on real problems. If you're anxious that a surgical procedure is dangerous, it probably is. If you're worried about the long-term side effects of a medication, you probably have good reason. In fact, as you make your own medical decisions, you'd be remiss if you didn't consider the consequences carefully. Your worries, therefore, aren't imaginary. They are compelling and should never be dismissed.

Some people fear that their feelings during this vulnerable time are "irrational." In truth, emotions are never rational or logical—they're emotions. Moreover, given the high state of anxiety that chronic illness provokes, it seems perfectly normal to feel irrational at this time. Emotions and actions are distinct, however. Feeling irrational does not mean that you'll act irrationally.

A final note: It's important to recognize that your worst fear may never come true. Since the course of most chronic illnesses is unpredictable, your situation could improve rather than worsen, as in the case of one distraught woman who had checked into the hospital to undergo risky surgery for the removal of a tumor in her neck. During the final pre-operative exam, her surgeon discovered that the tumor had shrunk and surgery was no longer necessary. Until that moment, it had never occurred to this woman that she would be spared the operation!

FIND A WAY TO RELEASE TENSION

Whether or not you try to hide from your fears, your feelings still come out, one way or another. Tension can vent itself inappropriately, as with a parent who yells at her child rather than her illness—the real source of her anger (see chapter 10 on misplaced anger). Even if the youngster's behavior is annoying or frustrating, the intensity of the reaction can indicate that the emotions have been misdirected.

It's good to relieve the pressure of intense emotion. Appropriate releases might include jogging, gardening (especially weed pulling), listening to music, taking a break, pounding on the piano, playing tennis, reading a book, wringing towels, talking to a friend, visualizing peaceful scenes, or meditating. You may express pent-up emotions either blatantly (by screaming while alone in your car or banging a fist on a table) or subtly (by crying softly or just staring off into space). When the feelings are intense, some people beat on a pillow. Hitting a mattress with a tennis racket makes a great sound! These last two suggestions are primitive and don't solve the problem but they do wonders for temporarily relieving tension. With time, the intensity will abate and you will be able to put your feelings into words again.

Releasing tension is essential to your survival; there are health implications if you don't. Remaining in a state of high stress requires physical energy, which is in short supply when you're ill. Many studies confirm that stress exacerbates physical symptoms of disease while stress reduction helps to ameliorate them.

To visualize the release of tension, picture yourself as a pot in which water has reached a rolling boil. In fact, the water is boiling so rapidly, the lid is riding on a head of steam. You need a way to safely lift the lid to release the pent-up pressure. Once you do, rather than losing control, you'll find yourself back in charge. Your mind will become calm and organized again. You will think clearly and once more be able to make good decisions.

IDENTIFY YOUR COPING STYLE

People gravitate toward two basic coping styles. Think of it as a continuum. At one end, you'll find confronters. They must ventilate openly or they feel like the boiling pot, ready to flip its lid. They can't wait to let their feelings out. At the other end are the avoiders. If they expose their emotions, they feel as if their pot has boiled over. They want desperately to keep the lid on. It's as stressful for the avoider to express his emotions as it is for the confronter to keep them in.

Actually, despite their tendency toward stoicism, avoiders still express their feelings. They just do so differently from confronters. When an avoider is upset, a few terse words and some quiet tears may accomplish for him what a deluge of emotionally charged paragraphs does for the confronter. It's a question of degree. Avoiders may have better control over their feelings or they may share the same feelings but with varying intensity. It's not necessarily true that confronters are stronger than avoiders or that it's better to talk than to keep feelings inside. In fact, sometimes, the opposite may be true.

It may help you to understand where you fit in the continuum. Once you recognize your style, you can make adjustments and accommodate to your family members' style of coping. The following exercise may help you identify how you deal with stress.

Imagine the following situations in which you're sure to be stressed:

1. Your twelve-year-old daughter went out to a new friend's house and promised to be back by 9 P.M. She neglected to leave the phone number and it's 10:30 now. (This is a short-term stress.)
2. Your spouse went to Los Angeles on a business trip for a couple of days. This morning your car was hit by a truck as you were taking your kids to school. Two of the children have broken bones and the car is totaled. (This is a crisis.)
3. You just took a routine stress test and the doctor told you not to play tennis this afternoon. (This is a medical crisis.)
4. You've discovered a lump in your breast (or in your testicle) and a test indicates that it might be cancerous. (This is a medical crisis.)
5. You've been experiencing stomachaches when you're pressured by deadlines and bottom lines and you think an ulcer may be developing. (This is a medical crisis.)

Now ask yourself the following questions for each situation and observe your reactions:

A. Do you sit down quietly and think about the best thing to do?
B. Do you call a family member and ask him or her for advice?
C. Do you feel panic?
D. Do you not know what to do?

E. Do you keep it to yourself?

F. Do you tell everyone of your concerns?

G. Do you laugh and make jokes?

H. Do you feel hungry? Do you reach for chocolate or raid the refrigerator?

I. Are you planning how you'll get through this?

J. Are you drawing a blank, hoping something will turn up?

If you've answered "yes" to questions D, E, G, H, and J for most of these situations, you tend toward being an avoider. And if you've answered "yes" to questions A, B, C, F, and I, you tend toward being a confronter. Even if your responses are mixed, you'll find that you come down more heavily either as a confronter or an avoider. Now, ask your family members to take the same quiz. How do they rate? Are their coping styles similar to yours or are they at the other end of the spectrum?

A word of caution: Once you understand and accept your coping style, be careful of extremes. Avoiders need to be careful not to become so inwardly focused that their suppressed feelings become physically harmful. Some form of self-expression, no matter how mild, such as telling one close friend once about how you feel, can be helpful. Conversely, if confronters share their feelings ad nauseam, they may sustain their own anxiety rather than relieve it. It's important to recognize one's limits. One young woman who couldn't stop expressing her feelings drove everyone, including strangers in my waiting room, away from her. At either extreme, you lose control!

It's also vital to recognize which coping styles you and your loved ones have adopted in order to judge whether you're coping in ways that are natural to you. Trying to behave in an alien manner can cause much suffering, since you'll be going against your nature. A "better" yet unfamiliar way of coping will not reduce stress but add to it.

I learned this lesson the hard way. As a confronter, I was used to expressing my feelings. With the advent of my children's severe illnesses, however, I feared losing control if I let out my emotions and so I kept them in for years, an unnatural state for me. One night, about a month before my daughter's second open heart surgery, however, I could no longer tolerate the pain.

My husband and I attended a symphony concert in an effort to stave off our anxiety. As I sat quietly in Constitution Hall, listening to the rise and swell of Beethoven's music, I was suddenly overcome with a nearly unsuppressible urge to scream. I could barely contain it and at the same time, I imagined the relief I would feel if I let out a blood-curdling shriek. But I also envisioned a small group of strongmen grabbing my wrists, strapping me into a straitjacket, and pushing me into an ambulance. My rational side knew this was impossible but the thought so terrified me that I ran out of the hall, my frightened husband at my heels.

Years later, in trying to understand this bizarre event, I realized I had been placing myself under inordinate stress by avoiding my feelings about my daughter's illness and particularly about her upcoming surgery. In one terrible moment, my mind had rebelled against all the years of bottled-up fears. I came within seconds of losing control because I had never expressed my anxiety and rage. I had not remained true to my innate coping style. After this incident, I never again tried to cope in a way alien to my personality.

In addition to identifying your own style, it's also important to recognize which style feels most comfortable to close family members. If a man who tends to confront his problems tries to force his wife, an avoider, to express her feelings, it could prove harmful to both. The reluctant wife could turn her unexpressed frustration and anger against her husband. Of course, the reverse is also true: one female confronter dragged her more reticent husband to support groups. The experience was wonderful for her, but it led him to ask for a divorce. A family member who has been forced into an unfamiliar coping style may feel as if he is making a personal sacrifice that cannot be maintained for the long haul.

If your spouse is reluctant to express emotions, don't push. Nevertheless, you can still explain that even though you understand his or her restraint, you need to cope by confronting your feelings. You may feel disappointed that your closest ally doesn't communicate the way you do, but don't underestimate your spouse's feelings. Even though the means of expression differs, they may be as strong as yours.

Aware of this disparity, you can seek help from others to satisfy your need for confrontation. You can find outlets at support groups, among friends, and with other extended family members.

APPRECIATE THAT ADJUSTMENT IS AN EBB AND FLOW

It's important to recognize that adjustment is not a continual forward movement, like a slow trek up the side of a mountain, but rather more like the ebb and flow of the tides. Most likely, in the course of coping with your illness, you'll experience fluctuating emotional states ranging from elation to depression and various levels of stress from mild discomfort to high anxiety. It is natural for your feelings to be in constant flux; adjustment is a long, difficult, and not particularly orderly process. If you understand and expect this movement, you won't feel disappointed when the tide turns.

One morning, you may awaken and, rather than fearing the day ahead, discover that you actually anticipate its pleasures. In place of the usual lassitude, you may experience a surge of energy. You may hesitate to formulate the thought, but still you chance it: "Has the tide turned? Will life be good again?" You spend the remainder of the day with shoulders held high—a weight has been lifted.

But that very evening, just as you're beginning to doze off, you may feel tingling slowly creeping up your arms and legs. You are frightened again. These are the symptoms of your illness or even extreme anxiety. Your wonderful day of feeling good has ended. Experiencing intense anger, you begin to blame yourself. "How did I cause this setback?" Reviewing your day, you find nothing that could have triggered the reappearance of symptoms. As the familiar helplessness returns, you bury your head in your pillow and cry silently but hard. You ask yourself again and again, "Why now?"

Remembering how wonderful your day was, you now feel as if you've struggled to the top of a mountain only to have your clutching fingers pried loose one at a time by some sinister being hiding in the dark behind the ledge. You fight to hang on to your good feelings, knowing how hard it was to reach them. Yet at the same time, you experience yourself sliding back down into despair. You'll have to climb this rocky path again. Your disappointment is deep.

This is the adjustment process. It's not a steady climb— no ten easy steps. Besides, since the course of many chronic illnesses is unpredictable, adjustment and accommodation today doesn't mean that you've conquered tomorrow's problems. If you buy into that, you'll constantly find yourself at the mercy of your illness. Catching you off guard, it will toss your emotions every which way as it veers from remission to recurrence and then back again. The trick is to cope with each situation as it occurs, no matter where it takes you. *If you expect the unexpectable, you—and not your illness—will be in charge of your life.*

Eventually adjustment does occur. You may be in your tenth struggle with your demon when one night you're blessed with an insight. You remember that you've fought off the darkness many times before; you even remember how you did it. You know that you've survived the tumble down and what it took to reach the pinnacle again. This is the point at which you realize you're living with your illness and that you can handle any anxiety it causes.

What got you through? In *Living with Cancer*, Dr. Ernest H. Rosenbaum calls this moment of insight "a flame of inner strength." He writes, "Call it what you will, the fear of dying, the will to live, or sheer determination, whatever it is, there is a toughness in all of us that makes us try again." Even when you feel the most despairing, have reached rock bottom, have no place to turn, you can still call upon an element of hope. Strange as it may sound, rock bottom has an advantage: from the depths, you can only go up!

It helps to remember that although today you're overwhelmed with anguish and heartache, you may feel better tomorrow. You might awaken one morning thinking your life is over—it will never be good again. And then two hours later, a friend calls and asks you to choose a movie—he'll be over at noon to pick you up. Suddenly the world seems brighter. How can you have such a reversal of feelings in so short a time? Your disease hasn't changed but your feelings about your life have! You're learning about adjustment and integration.

INTEGRATION

When you have integrated your chronic disease, you realize that the bitter medicine that had made you gag no longer upsets your stomach. In fact, this unpleasant ritual has even become routine. Other reminders of your illness no longer dominate your thinking, just as they elude those diabetic or epileptic marathon runners who, despite their diseases, are impossible to distinguish in a crowd.

Even though the changes caused by your illness are difficult and painful, you can adjust to them. The process is neither easy nor orderly but if your coping style matches your
personality, you'll keep stress to a minimum. You are intact,
you can cope, and you can once again be in charge of your life.

REMEMBER

- Since chronic illness is different from any you've experienced previously, you'll be coping differently too.
- Understand the complexity of your current situation:
you're like a pane of glass that has been hit very hard;
the glass may be cracked but it's still whole.
- Face your fears. They are valid. Nevertheless, the
worst of them may never come true.
- It's important to relieve tension. Find the way that's
best for you.
- Recognize and respect your own coping style and that
of your loved ones. You're each entitled to deal with
the medical crisis in your own way. Don't force your
style on someone else and don't allow others to impose
their style on you. Watch for extremes.
- Feelings change. Those that are overpowering today
may be only a vague memory tomorrow. Adjustment is
not an orderly process.
- Your medical condition is unpredictable and so your
emotions may swing widely as your condition alters.
- People who integrate their disease find it no longer
dominates their lives.

3.

Family Members: Making the Most of Changing Relationships

After the diagnosis or onset of a long-term illness, your relationship with your family will inevitably change. You may want extra attention and they may feel burdened by new responsibilities. Besides, just as you cannot deny being overwhelmed by the many problems you face, so can you not deny that your family faces them with you—their future is tied to yours. This is a time of high anxiety for all of you, when even the closest bonds and the best of family relations may become strained. Nevertheless, understanding the potential for family breakdown can give you the power to prevent it.

THE NEAR BREAKDOWN OF A FAMILY

Paul, a father of two children who lived in Bethesda, had been diagnosed with multiple sclerosis in his twenties but suffered few effects until he was in his late forties. He had always been a handsome, virile, and athletic man. As a bright and successful real estate broker, he had found his work satisfying and financially rewarding.

However, due to the worsening of his condition over the last several years, Paul had evolved from an optimistic go-getter into an extremely angry person. I was aware of this from the moment he walked into my office. His lips were white with tension and his piercing brown eyes glared at his surroundings. Indeed, the room almost vibrated with his rage.

Moreover, his wife, Marilyn, was equally upset, as were their children (ages nine and eleven), who consequently experienced difficulties in school. In truth, although Paul was the identified patient, all four members of this family were deeply affected by multiple sclerosis. A neurologist had referred Paul and his family to me to help them deal with their trauma.

As I began to treat this family, I discovered that Paul had always vented his emotions loudly and clearly, no matter what effect his behavior had had on those around him. Marilyn, on the other hand, accepted her emotions quietly. She was forever sensitive about hurting other's feelings.

When Paul was healthy, the couple had adjusted to this disparity. But as Paul became increasingly debilitated he began to experience the eight fears so common in people diagnosed with chronic illnesses. As he became more and more dependent on Marilyn's care, his anger grew by leaps and bounds. He avoided his friends and colleagues, fearing that they looked down on him now that he was handicapped, and he worried that his family would ultimately abandon him to the care of a nursing home. He feared that his life was whirling out of control. Ashamed of his disabilities and dependency, he vented his feelings by criticizing his accepting wife and belittling her mistakes and fears.

Paul's escalating irascibility became intolerable for Marilyn in her more vulnerable state. As a result of his psychologically abusive behavior, she felt herself on the verge of suicide. Although she managed her husband's physical care quite efficiently, and even felt gratified by it, she could no longer endure his verbal assaults. Every time he railed at her about how inadequate she was at performing a task that he believed he had been better equipped to handle before he became ill, she wanted to crawl into a hole and die.

Clearly, this family was bordering on disintegration when they came to see me. I helped them to adjust to the changes that multiple sclerosis had brought into their lives. In particular, I worked with them on their communication, since continuing their existing patterns would have been destructive to them and their marriage. Neither spouse wanted divorce; they wished to stay together as a family. Paul loved Marilyn deeply and enjoyed his wife's attention. For her part, Marilyn wanted to continue caring for her husband.

During our sessions, I helped each of them understand how the other felt. Paul realized that he appreciated his wife and didn't want to hurt her, while Marilyn learned to ask for and get the respite she so desperately needed.

The goals of this chapter are to help you to appreciate and respect your own emotions, to help you become aware of and understand your family's feelings (as Paul and Marilyn did), and to help the members of your family communicate as many of these sentiments as possible within a context of loving acceptance. When you eliminate the barriers to communication, you will be taking steps to keep your family intact, despite the changes wrought by your disease. But first, let us take a closer look at why and how family relations can crumble as a result of chronic illnesses, especially since you will cope differently with your problems than the rest of your family.

WHY FAMILY COMMUNICATION CAN BECOME BLOCKED

Let's face it. Everyone is affected by your disease: your spouse, children, parents, grandparents, and even your grandchildren. Of course, your family will not experience the physical effects of your illness as you do, but they will certainly struggle with the same emotional, practical, and financial difficulties.

It may be hard for you to accept that your family is suffering along with you. You may feel somehow responsible. In fact you may experience a wide range of contradictory emotions from guilt, neediness, and rage to gratitude and ambivalence. But because of your feeling of responsibility, I believe it essential for you to understand that you are not the cause of your family's pain. Rather, your disease—an unwelcome intruder into all of your lives—is the culprit.

It may come as a surprise to you that your family might be more depressed and upset than you are! While you (and everyone else) expect them to be physically and emotionally strong—after all, they're well—in reality they are wrestling with the same eight fears of long-term illness that have complicated your life. They too feel out of control, stigmatized, and isolated. They are angry and find their self-image challenged. They feel inadequate to handle your care and perhaps your new emotional dependency. They are deeply ashamed because they sometimes wish they could run away from the problem, making you fear their abandonment. The very act of considering the possibility of your death often leads them to confront the idea of their own mortality for the first time.

You should also be aware that the period immediately following your diagnosis or the onset of your illness is one of extreme anxiety for all of you because of these very fears and adversities. Consequently, this is a time fraught with the danger of family friction and breakdown. Just when you need each other the most, you may find yourselves at one another's throats. Or, worse yet, you may have stopped communicating altogether. Not that you don't converse—you still talk about everyday household management problems— but you no longer share your deepest feelings regarding what's upsetting you or your mutual needs for support.

Moreover, you may want to confide your emotions but may fear that once spoken, they will be misunderstood. This apprehension is not so farfetched. Families consist of a system of interdependencies: what affects one member affects the whole. Since all of the people in your family are integrally involved with one another, it's difficult for any of you to be objective.

The issues that are the most frightening for you may also be the most frightening for your mate. Misunderstandings and the loss of intimacy are common at this time. For example, after having been diagnosed with lung cancer, Judith wanted to talk about her fear of dying. Her husband, Barry, couldn't bear the thought and so cut her off in mid-sentence whenever she broached the subject. Unfortunately, Judith misinterpreted her husband's avoidance. She took it to mean that he didn't love her, while in truth he was only trying to save his own sanity.

Men often have a harder time sharing their emotions. Society has taught them that they must control their feelings, and so they're afraid that if they give in to them, they'll fall apart and lose their ability to work and function. Women are frequently better equipped to listen to their spouses than men. In fact, I have seen that sometimes men tune out their wives. This doesn't mean that they love their spouses less or are avoiding them. Rather, it's an indication that they simply can't express their emotions in words. (If a woman with an unreceptive husband needs to talk with someone, she should find a friend, relative, or counselor to confide in.)

Finally, you are all facing something new. In the past, your family may have been plagued by external problems. You had learned that by banding together and cooperating or rallying around the person in trouble, you were able to reach some resolution. With the advent of a chronic illness, however, the "enemy" (in the guise of the disease) is within. The whole family shares a common destiny that requires all of you to adjust.

THE CONSEQUENCES OF THE COMMUNICATION GAP

The lack of meaningful dialogue can devastate your family, much as it had Paul and Marilyn's. While some individuals, like Paul, use anger to deflect important discussions, others use avoidance. You may all repress emotions deemed unacceptable, causing you and your family to express them indirectly, ineffectually, and perhaps even destructively. The consequences can be disastrous, since loved ones may withdraw from you or may become hostile just when you're the most vulnerable.

In order to sidestep talking about unpleasant or painful topics, your relations may begin avoiding *you*. They may withdraw subtly and unconsciously for fear of bringing up those subjects they fear would hurt you. For instance, one of my patients, Ella, realized that her husband had been staying at his office later and later each night; he sometimes even went into work on the weekends. And Paula suddenly left her husband's bedside and started to visit her sick cousin three nights a week. Her abrupt absence just when her husband needed her most left him wondering, "Why now?"

If the verbal avenues of communication have become gridlocked, you and your family may find other, less effective means of venting your powerful emotions. You may all believe, for example, that you have put your feelings on hold. This is an illusion. In reality these powerful emotions lie quiescent, just waiting for any opportunity (appropriate or not) to surface.

They may emerge, for example, when your husband casually reminds you that you forgot to take your morning medication. This innocent act can trigger a stream of invective that leaves him in an astonished silence, wondering, "What did I say to provoke that outburst?" Or on the way to a vacation, your wife may suddenly thrust your wheelchair onto a fast-moving airport escalator, absolutely terrifying you. "Isn't she pushing this wheelchair extra hard?" you ask yourself. In these instances, you may be confronted with loved ones' strong feelings of anger that they have been unwilling or unable to verbalize.

WHAT FAMILY MEMBERS MAY BE THINKING

In my years as a medical crisis counselor, I've discovered that communication can improve and that relationships can and do mend when patients and their families have a look behind the scenes at one another's thoughts and feelings. Let's bring these issues into focus in order to help you and your loved ones open a meaningful dialogue.

You may be surprised to learn, for example, that in some ways you have an easier time psychologically than your loved ones. Why? To begin with, your spouse may be burdened with guilt that he's not doing enough to help you. Moreover, he may feel ashamed of his feelings and fears. He may believe that you are entitled to be upset but that he isn't. He may feel more isolated than you and close to burnout. Indeed, if he feels backed into a corner, he may run, which will only exacerbate his negative self-image. I have often found that the ill individual has a better handle on his or her emotions than does the spouse!

What are some of the other thoughts going on inside the heads of those closest to you? I have gathered the following helpful, albeit painful list of feelings from my experience counseling family members of the chronically ill:

- They may feel angry and resentful because plans for future education, travel, weddings, vacation, or retirement must now be delayed or canceled.
- They may feel shame when they're out with you and people stare at your wheelchair, cane, or ungainly gait. Then they feel guilty for the shame. (After all, you love one another. How could they be ashamed about the way you look?)
- They worry about their own health when they become tired or depressed. If they become ill, they brood about who will pick up the responsibility for your care, both physical and financial.
- When they fret about their health, they feel guilty because you're the one who's "really" sick and suffering.
- They urge you to take better care of yourself and feel guilty because their sentiments aren't entirely altruistic: they're tired of the responsibility and wish to lighten their own burden.
- They resent that you sometimes take advantage of your illness to manipulate them, but fearing that they'll upset you and aggravate your symptoms, they remain silent.

Even while maintaining a difficult silence, family members may wish that they could do more for you. Yet, in today's mobile society, families are smaller and extended families have scattered far and wide. In fact, doing more may become an increasingly difficult task without adequate support. Your small nuclear family may still wish to provide the kind of care they feel you deserve, but loved ones have no fresh troops to call in when they feel exhausted. Often, the spouse is the major if not only caregiver. Yet, from the many families I have seen, I know that it is virtually impossible for one person totally to fulfill another's physical, emotional, and financial needs. Unrealistic expectations on both sides can lead to deep disappointments and the caregiver's burnout.

It's also important for you to recognize that your family may have reached a different level of acceptance than you. For example, you may be beginning to achieve a sort of peace with your illness—"What will be, will be"—whereas your family may still be searching for the ultimate cure. Thinking that you have lost faith, they may feel responsible for keeping hope alive. In truth, you are facing reality, but they are not.

Finally, you must realize that you are getting far more support from doctors, nurses, clergy, other family members, and friends than your caregivers may receive. Often, they are left to struggle alone. And even if friends offer them support, they may feel undeserving of it because they aren't the "sick" one in the family. Like you, they need support. Paul's wife, Marilyn, said, "You know, I can manage almost anything if I just get a few words of encouragement from my husband and kids."

WHAT YOU MAY BE THINKING

Just as you need to understand what your loved ones feel toward you, you must now examine your feelings toward them. Your emotions may be even more frightening and intense than theirs. Even if you could articulate them, you may be afraid of being misunderstood, so you remain silent. What's more, you may believe that your family is overwhelmed already and you have no desire to add to their burden.

I have compiled the following list, gleaned from my practice, to help you identify your own emotions. If you read with an objective eye, you will notice that many individuals suffering from long-term illnesses express ambivalent feelings; these can be destructive because they convey mixed messages to the family. Although these statements may be difficult to read, understanding how you feel will eventually help you air your emotions with your kin:

- You feel that your family can never understand you because they're not sick, but you desperately wish that they could.
- You are annoyed every time your family asks you how you're feeling; you want them to know without their having to ask.
- You're envious of their good health and physical strength, but you worry that if they become too tired, they will be unable to care for you.
- You dislike being treated as a child, but you feel a sense of relief to know someone can take care of you as needed.
- You long for intimacy and warmth, but sometimes wish to be left alone when you're tired.
- You feel put off when your spouse says, "We'll talk about your chemotherapy treatment schedule tomorrow," but relieved because you weren't eager to discuss it either.
- You worry whether your husband or wife finds you attractive in your new condition, but you neglect to spruce up your appearance for when he or she comes home from work.
- You fear being unloved but imagine that you are unlovable in your new, "flawed" state.

In addition, you may wish to express your frustration, anger, and hopelessness without a two-way conversation. You may not want to hear how your spouse is tired and tied down. What you actually want is a warm, sympathetic ear. You long to hear words of unconditional compassion and support—the kind you might have received from a parent when you were feeling vulnerable and frightened. Indeed, you may *say* that you want to listen to your spouse's feelings, but it may be too hurtful to know that he is suffering because of your illness—a situation over which you have neither power nor control. In truth all you really want are expressions of love and steadfast devotion.

You must also anticipate that you may never be able to express some feelings to your loved ones and that you can expect friction because of that. One of my patients, Shirley, had a strong need to talk with her husband about her fear of dying after a bout with breast cancer. But Irving simply couldn't discuss this with her. In fact, her pressing him to relate on this level only made him withdraw more. While Shirley had been considering the implications of her illness (including death) for a long time, Irving had considered them quickly and then removed them from his conscious mind because they were too painful.

I advised Shirley to turn to another resource, such as her brother, sister, or aunt. I also reminded her that although she wanted to talk with her husband, the more subtle ways of communicating—cuddling, holding hands, and exchanging meaningful looks—might speak volumes.

PUTTING THE PROBLEM IN PERSPECTIVE

Even in your present state of vulnerability, you do have the power to help yourself and your family. Rather than allowing the continuing disintegration of your relationships, when you take charge, you can help bring everyone together. You can avoid separation, divorce, and even institutionalization. The very first step is to put your problems into perspective. It may be helpful to ask yourself the following questions:

- What were my family relations like before this illness?
- How did my family cope with mutual problems before it struck?
- Is this the most serious problem we've all faced together?
- How have my losses affected my family? What have they lost as a result of my illness?
- Has our social life changed? How about our work life?
- Has this illness given me the opportunity to improve my family relations, or has it made them worse?

Next, realize that *the cause of your difficulties is your illness, not you.* All of you must understand this fact. You must come to accept that you have not precipitated this disease—*you are not at fault.* Even though you know you could have exercised more, drank less coffee, or left an extremely stressful job, even though your family warned you to change your behavior or your life-style and you ignored them, your disease may be a result of your genetic history or another completely unknown—or unknowable— factor.

So, while you or they may *feel* as if you have brought this problem on yourself, the truth is most likely you have not. Certain individuals are predisposed to particular illnesses and science has not yet figured out why. On the other hand, some people smoke heavily all their lives and never get lung cancer. Others rarely exercise and eat ice cream daily and somehow avoid heart disease. We are just beginning to understand how gene pools influence disease. Blaming yourself is counterproductive.

ADJUST YOUR EXPECTATIONS

Even when you're not sick, marriage is a matter of give and take. The advent of your illness will cause you to reassess and adjust your expectations of your loved ones because your relationship will probably be thrown off kilter. Ask yourself the following questions:

- Who are the "givers" and "takers" in my family?
- Where do I fit in?
- Can I expect this situation to change? (Some people are natural givers while others are not, but want to be. They may love you but may need your guidance on how to be helpful.)
- Has the balance of give and take shifted as a result of my diagnosis? How? In what direction?
- Are my parents able to give more to me than my spouse or children? Why?
- If I'm a giver, is it hard for me to take? If I'm a taker, can I be asking too much of my caregiver?
- What can I expect from each person closest to me?
- Is it tenable to expect unconditional support? If so, from whom? (Be realistic.)

Perhaps your spouse has less tolerance for personal pain than you do. Perhaps she lacks the ability to handle the extra responsibilities that your illness requires. Be patient with your family as members assume new roles like driving a van or handling the budget, the cooking, or the family business. Your loved ones may be doing less than you had hoped but chances are this is the best they can muster at this time. Not only do they not have the experience, but they may also feel intimidated and anxious. They need your support. Respect the individual differences among you and be realistic about energy levels and abilities.

Don't be disappointed if you're not the family's constant center of attention; you need their concern, not their lives. Besides, yours may not be the only problem they are facing. Your son may be having marital difficulties or your wife may be suffering back problems. They may need your support as they attempt to cope with their own issues.

You may wish so, but you should not expect that your family will be able to read your mind. You must tell your loved ones how you feel and what you're needing in order for a frank exchange to occur and for your needs to be met. This is not easy. You may be unsure of what you want from them, or you may be afraid that you're asking too much. You would prefer that they be forthcoming with little effort on your part.

BREAKING OUT OF YOUR ISOLATION

Taking charge means initiating open communication with your family regarding your illness and all of its ramifications. You may feel as if this is a responsibility you don't want or need. After all, you have enough to worry about already. On the other hand, you are also the one with the most to lose if a frank dialogue does not occur. If your caregivers remain uninformed of your needs, you may feel neglected. Your brave front can hide more than you realize. In fact, your family may believe that they are required to do less because you seem so self-contained.

Look at it this way. You understand your feelings better than anyone else. Without a frame of reference, your family may be unable to read your emotions or your behavior. Unless they understand you, you cannot expect them to help you in the ways you feel you need to be helped. Therefore, it is incumbent upon you to let them know exactly how you feel.

COMMUNICATION SKILLS
THAT CAN HELP

In opening communications, it's important to proceed cautiously, since inappropriately expressed feelings can give rise to big arguments. If you communicate appropriately, you can help bring your family closer together. The following suggestions may help:

1. Arrange a quiet time. Schedule a date to talk with your family about matters relating to your health. This will give you all time to consider the issues. Make sure other appointments don't interfere. Unless someone is expecting an urgent call, let your answering machine pick up your phone messages.

2. Sit down. It helps if you are all on the same physical and emotional level. Your loved ones will feel they are on an equal footing and will believe you'll really listen to one another if you take the time to sit down and discuss your issues in a focused way.

3. Explain clearly. When you begin communicating, don't mince words or couch your emotions in half-truths. For example, avoid saying "You seem to have your head in a book all the time," when you really mean "I feel neglected." If your family misunderstands your first attempts at explaining yourself, try a second or third time. Use other words and examples such as "I feel vulnerable right now and need extra support." Whatever you do, be sure to get your point across. (See more about making "I" statements on page 208.)

It's best to ask if you've made yourself clear. You can even request confirmation by saying "What did you hear me say?" If your listener has misconstrued your words, correct him by saying, "No, this is what I meant."

4. *Really listen.* You may have a lot on your mind, but you need to pay attention to what your family members have to say too. Listening is an active form of communication. A person who is listened to feels cared about and valued. Listening implies mutual respect. All of you will need to feel listened to in order for your dialogue to be successful. If a family member cuts you off in midthought, remind her that you heard her out when it was her turn to speak; now it's only fair that she listen to you too.

If after listening, you feel you've been misinterpreted, you might say "You're not hearing me." It's hard to break through the barriers of defenses that we set up, so try again. Do speak in a calm voice and explain yourself in a different way.

5. *Make eye contact.* Poets have called the eyes the windows to the soul. Emotions, especially love, are expressed through the eyes. From earliest infancy onward, we all understand these nonverbal cues. When you look into your loved one's eyes, you are letting him know that your attention is focused on him and him alone.

If a family member has the tendency to cast his eyes downward, you can gently remind him that you find it hard to know what he's feeling inside if he's staring at the floor. You can say "I'm afraid I may miss what you're trying to tell me."

If he still can't look you in the eye, tell him "It's OK. I understand why you have difficulty looking me straight in the eye." Perhaps as you continue your discussion, he will come around. Never force the other person to do what he does not want to do.

6. *Ask questions in nonthreatening ways.* Expressions such as "How come you always . . . ?" or "Why don't you ever . . . ?" are the stuff that power struggles are made of, and nobody wins a power struggle. These statements cause your loved ones to become defensive, and that works against

your best interest. It's preferable to approach difficult situations with an element of curiosity in your voice. You can say "Help me understand what's going on with you, Maria. I'm feeling lonely and miss having you around. I really want to know how you feel. Please help me." By telling Maria how *you* feel, you give her permission to reveal how *she* feels. Keep your voice as calm as possible. This opens the way for your discussion about your relationship.

You really must understand how your family member is feeling. If you don't, keep asking in different ways until you do. If you achieve only partial understanding, explain which areas are clear to you and which are not. If you can't accomplish understanding in one meeting, try again the next time you meet.

If you feel angry, wait until the intensity has diminished before you speak.

7. *Use mirroring.* The technique of mirroring validates your loved one's emotional experience by communicating *your* understanding of what *he* is feeling. You can say, for example, "Brett, I can see that you're upset about missing that fishing trip next week. I know you were looking forward to it for a long time and it's important to you." By mirroring your family member's emotions, you show him that you understand and respect him. Consequently, you will set the tone for how your family copes.

8. *Give your family permission for their feelings.* Your family will undoubtedly experience feelings of anxiety and inadequacy in caring for you. You can eliminate some of their guilt (especially when they're tired and angry) by giving them permission to feel the way they do. You can say, for example, "I understand that you feel overwhelmed by my care. It's taking a lot out of you. You're tired and frustrated."

Even quite negative feelings are normal at this time, so be prepared for them. You can expect to feel hurt, but if you tolerate these emotions and recognize that they're directed at the situation and not at you, you'll be able to understand your loved one and he'll feel appreciated.

If it helps your family, let them know that you have negative feelings too. For example, you may wish to share with them that you are jealous of their good health and new-found ability to fulfill family responsibilities that were once yours. (But also let them know that you need them to take care of themselves so they can be strong for you!) When you give your family permission for their feelings, they will be more open with you.

9. Separate your loved one from her actions. In order to keep your family member's self-esteem intact, it's important to distinguish between the person and her behavior. Focus on the act, rather than the individual. If you say "Heather, I love you, but I feel hurt when you make faces every time I ask you to take me to the doctor. I already feel guilty for your having to do this," you communicate that you continue to value your daughter, even though you find her behavior difficult to accept.

Stick with *your* emotions. Rather than attacking your family member's character, it's more acceptable to say that you feel hurt, angry, or frustrated. This keeps your relative from becoming defensive.

10. Examine your own emotions. You can distort and express with great anger feelings that you misunderstand. For example, if your husband's desire to attend a basketball game with his pals makes you furious, you might blurt out in rage, "You just can't wait to get away from me, can you?"

On the other hand, if you can be more honest about your feelings toward your caregiver, you will be more sensitive to his—and less demanding too. You can do this without expressing your emotions openly. Talk to yourself. Say "I know he needs a break. I'm afraid to be left alone for a few hours, but I *can* manage. I'm angry that he wants to go to a basketball game with his buddies. Why am I angry? Because I can't go? Because I'm jealous? That's not his doing."

Then, you can say out loud to your spouse "I'm jealous that I can't go. I wish I could, but it's important for you to get out. You've been very good to me." In this way, you will resolve your conflict more readily.

11. Keep your antenna tuned to unspoken communication. Facial expressions, body language, and even silence all communicate some feelings, which need to be understood and articulated. Give your spouse respite. She may need the opportunity to process all that you've said. Silence can be calming.

12. Express love. Love is ongoing; anger is temporary. Despite the angry feelings that may be aired during your discussion, it's best to find some way to express your underlying feelings of love and caring for one another. This will cement your relationship despite the difficulties you all share. After all, you are still the same people you were before the illness struck.

FEELINGS YOU MIGHT WANT TO SHARE

You may believe that your family cannot understand you because they're not sick. I have found, however, that although they can't identify with you completely, they can be supportive if you let them know what you're thinking. You might want to share the following emotions and needs with your family to spur open communication:

- Tell them that you don't expect them to solve your problems. You just need them to listen and be supportive.
- Tell them that you feel like a burden on them and need reassurance that they don't mind giving the extra attention you require.
- Tell them that you know they sometimes feel trapped by the illness and by you.
- Tell them that you have thought a lot about it and often feel the same way they do: you are all victims of your disease and the position it has put you in.
- Describe to them the kinds of support you need from them. If you want space and time alone, ask for it. If you need them to be around more, ask for that too. (This may not always work perfectly but it's better than not expressing your desires.)
- Let them know that you miss going places (like sporting events or concerts) with them that have become difficult for you to manage. Help them find alternative activities you can all enjoy or if you are too incapacitated to attend an event, encourage them to go with someone else.
- Tell them that you understand that they're not angry at you, but at the situation, so they need not feel guilty.
- Reassure them that you understand their feelings—they aren't too different from yours. You're in this together.
- Guide them on how to treat you: with sympathy, empathy, or support while honoring your independence and your feelings.
- Let them know how important they are to you. You need them and you need to be needed.
- Tell them how much you appreciate all that they're doing for you, even if they can't meet your expectations. (In fact, given the circumstances, you might have to reevaluate those expectations.)
- Ask how they feel about talking about your illness; do they fear being hurtful toward you? What subjects does it

hurt them to bring up and what ones are all right to bring up? (Be sensitive about how much they can tolerate.)
- Ask if you're being unreasonably demanding. Back off if you are!
- Ask if they need time off. If they do, tell them that you understand their needs and want them to have respite.

Watch for the danger signs of burnout, such as withdrawal and short tempers or anger directed at you. You can suggest family counseling if you feel that tension is building and you don't know how to handle it. A minister or rabbi, hot-line volunteer, self-help group, good friend, or professional counselor can help in times of difficulty.

HELPING YOUR FAMILY ADJUST TO CHANGING RESPONSIBILITIES

The advent of your illness may have created a shift in responsibilities, causing you and your family to adapt to unaccustomed roles. Your wife may find herself suddenly having to take over as the family's chief wage earner, or your husband may find himself saddled with unfamiliar household chores.

Moreover, you may feel resentful that you are being displaced. Suddenly you have been robbed of your importance in the family. This change in roles is significant. It can mean your giving up control, a loss of your identity, and a change in your self-image. It's not easy! While you're feeling resentful, your family members may be nervous about taking on new and difficult tasks. It's plain to see how feelings can be hurt.

But here too by taking charge, you can facilitate your family's adjustment.

1. Keep as much responsibility as you can handle. You may feel inclined to turn over all of your responsibilities to your family (see chapter 5 on becoming passive). It's wise, however, to keep as many family jobs as you can because that helps you retain your sense of self-worth and your value to your family. When you're pulling your own weight in the group, you will engender your family's respect and, most important, your own.

2. Maintain your responsibility over medical decisions. Making your own medical decisions helps you to preserve your integrity and control over your life (see chapter 5). It also eases your family's burden.

3. Watch for your family's overprotectiveness. If your loved ones are having difficulties with the hospital staff, try to be a link between the two factions. You may understand why the staff is behaving in a particular way whereas your family may not. Often, when families become overprotective, doctors and nurses perceive them as being intrusive (see chapter 4). If you find that your family is behaving in this way, decide how dependent you want to be. You may need to tell them that simply being supportive is the best help they can offer you. And you can offer to explain the two "factions" to each other—no one needs more stress at this time!

4. Don't take advantage of your family's guilt. Some people who crave attention use their illness to the point of abusing their families. If your loved ones feel sorry for you, you must be careful not to use their emotions manipulatively. Be responsible about your demands, even while you like the extra attention.

5. *Arrange for and welcome respite for your caregivers.*
Watch for the signs of burnout and remember that it's not a
permanent state. Burnout simply lets you know that your
family needs time to recoup. When you freely and willingly
"give" your loved ones time off, you lessen their guilt.
Besides, you really don't want them to sneak off to a movie
or dinner—that's demeaning and demoralizing for them and
may make them angry at you for causing them to feel that
way. The whole family will benefit if your loved ones maintain their own physical and mental health.

LOOKING ON THE BRIGHT SIDE

Your disease may have caused you to be an added responsibility to your family, but that doesn't mean you're a burden. Often, illnesses act as catalysts, bringing the family
closer together. Some of the happiest times for families
occur when members share and conquer mutual problems,
when they must cooperate to benefit you and themselves.

Looking back on the many families I've treated, I have
found that even though these individuals may have struggled painfully, sometimes for years, ultimately what they
recall are the positive aspects of the illness. Values change
for the better. Caregiving becomes gratifying—an act of
love. You spend more time together, pleasing one another.
One family, for example, took great pains to help their ill
father attend regular hockey games, despite his disabilities.
They took pleasure in renting a van and transporting him
en masse. Families do survive chronic illness intact.

REMEMBER

- You and your family share this problem.
- This is a time of high anxiety; even the best family
  relations are tested.

- Understanding the potential for family breakdown gives you the power to prevent it.
- You will cope differently from the members of your family.
- Your illness—and not you—is the cause of the stress.
- You and your family may have hidden feelings that you find difficult to share.
- Open the lines of communication, using appropriate skills.
- Watch for signals of burnout and discuss your mutual expectations for your care.
- Remain as responsible as possible for your own life.

THINGS TO DO

- Hand your family this book. Write notes in the margins for them to see.
- Set the tone for communication.
- Expect friction. It's normal.
- Communicate nonverbally by hugging and touching.
- Get an objective third person to mediate if you run into trouble.
- Give your family time off; they'll appreciate it.
- Be patient as your spouse learns new roles.
- Work out leisure time and activities so that you don't feel abandoned and your loved ones don't feel trapped.
- Be a good companion. You may have lost certain assets but can develop others.
- Show your family how important they are to you and be valuable to them.
- Think about what you can do to help your family.

4.

Forging an Effective Doctor-Patient Partnership

Forging effective doctor-patient partnerships may be one of the most important "take charge" tools at your disposal. Over the course of your disease, your relationship with your physician will affect your emotional and personal well-being, not just your physical condition. Your level of stress will decrease if you trust, respect, and feel comfortable with your physician; if you believe that he cares about you and will be responsive to you. Indeed, your interactions with your doctor will influence the quality of your daily activities and can affect life-and-death decisions. These are relationships that you should not underestimate, especially since your doctor may be caring for you for the rest of your life!

In this chapter, I'll provide backstage information to help you navigate the new maze of physicians, specialists, hospitals, nurses, and other health care professionals you're bound to encounter as a result of your disease. It is my hope that this will encourage you to be a responsive and responsible medical consumer—an active partner in the maintenance of your health.

"Oh God," you may be thinking. "As if I didn't have enough to worry about already! Between my illness and its effect on me and my family, I feel overwhelmed. And now I have to deal with this intimidating world of medicine. How am I going to cope?"

Rest assured. You can create supportive relationships with your physicians. When you establish the boundaries of your partnership early on, your doctor will be concerned with your feelings, not just your physical condition. That's important because your emotional comfort level with your doctor can affect how you respond to prescribed treatments. But first you must understand how your chronic condition differs from other medical problems you might have encountered in the past, and how your care will diverge too.

HOW LONG-TERM CARE
DIFFERS FROM ACUTE CARE

If, at some other point in your lifetime, you have suffered from an acute illness such as appendicitis or pneumonia, you may have met with your surgeon or doctor several times; she probably gave you a prompt diagnosis and administered treatment. Within a short period, you got better. Indeed, the diagnosis was clear and the recovery predictable and sure. You might never have needed to see that surgeon or doctor again. End of story.

With a long-term illness, on the other hand, your general practitioner will most likely refer you to a specialist. You may find that this new doctor seems more impersonal and colder than your GP. You should remember that unlike your GP, the specialist may know a lot about your body but little about you personally. In fact, she may have chosen to become a specialist to avoid deep personal relationships with patients.

Your first encounters with the specialist may be marked by frustration. For example, she may be unable to reach a clear diagnosis or may accurately analyze the problem only after exhaustive tests. Indeed, the waiting period between your first appointment with the specialist and a definitive diagnosis may seem like a special kind of purgatory. Your anxiety will most likely heighten as you undergo physically unpleasant or even risky tests. You may exhaust yourself from the constant worrying but still have to pay the mounting bills and fill out endless insurance forms.

Finally, your doctor will arrive at a definitive diagnosis. You may feel somewhat relieved that you now have something concrete to deal with, but the news isn't all that good. The specialist, for example, may have few options to offer as treatments. She may also explain that you will experience only an incomplete recovery; the progress of your disease may be unpredictable and unsure. Rather than a simple problem and solution so common with acute illnesses, your long-term condition may be fraught with ambiguities. The only certainty is that it cannot be cured.

ASKING THE RIGHT QUESTIONS

Despite the unwelcome news, you need not feel helpless with your physician or your illness. One of the best ways to take charge of your disease is to know exactly what you're dealing with. Unless you know what your disease is, how it manifests itself, its likely prognosis, and how the treatments may or may not help you, you cannot make a realistic evaluation of your medical condition or the course of action you should pursue. Indeed, unless you are fully informed, you cannot be responsible and in control of your medical decisions. That means asking the specialist the right questions.

Get as much information about your disease as is possible (although only as much as you're comfortable with at any given session). You may find the doctor-patient questions below helpful. These suggestions are intended to prod your thinking—your personal list will depend on your particular illness and your current physical condition. It may help you to write down your questions and bring them into your meeting with your doctor so you won't have to worry about forgetting what you wanted to ask.

- Are you sure of the diagnosis?
- How did I get this disease?
- What factors make it worse or better?
- How long must I stay in the hospital?
- What should I expect as far as disabilities? Will the disease get worse?
- Can the symptoms be controlled?
- What treatments are available?
- Is the treatment you're recommending the latest?
- What is its success rate?
- What are the risks of this treatment?
- Do the benefits outweigh the risks?
- Are there any experimental treatments I should know about?
- If I take this medication for many years, what are the potential side effects?
- If I have surgery, will it stop the disease or will the process continue?
- What should I be doing to take care of myself?
- What would make me feel better?
- What would make me feel worse?

- Is there anything I can do to slow the disease's progress?
- Will I have to limit my home activities and life-style?
- What kind of emotional reactions can I expect?
- What can I expect for the future?

These questions are general, but your physician and her staff should be willing to listen to you and to be forthcoming in their responses.

You may also wish to bring your spouse, a close relative, or friend along to ask questions that might have eluded you. Take notes (or ask your friend to take notes) during this important visit. The doctor may impart too much information for you to absorb all at once in your state of anxiety, and you'll want an extra pair of ears to help you hear and record everything.

If you don't understand an explanation, ask the physician to explain the disease in another way, without the medical jargon. You can say, for example, "I don't understand these terms. Could you use words I do understand?" Sometimes it's helpful if she can show you a three-dimensional model or draw a picture of the problem.

Even with a prepared list, you may not ask everything you want to know at a single appointment. You will be nervous, and new concerns might arise after you've had a chance to consider the information. A good doctor knows this. Your specialist and her staff must be willing to take your phone calls, as long as you don't make unreasonable demands on their time. Indeed, as you leave, ask if you can call later should other questions arise.

You might feel tempted to seek the specialist's advice regarding personal decisions, such as what you ought to do about your job, where you should live, or whether you should get married. These questions will most likely be difficult for your doctor to discuss, particularly because she doesn't know you well. For answers to queries such as these, you are perhaps better advised to talk with your general practitioner, who is more acquainted with you and your family situation.

Although your specialist will be your prime source of medical information, you may also wish to seek information about your illness from other sources:

- Use the public library. You may find books on your illness written for the layperson.
- National health organizations such as the American Cancer Society and the American Heart Association publish excellent brochures and pamphlets written by doctors and patients. Many of these organizations have toll-free numbers you can call for up-to-the-minute information.
- If you desire more technical information, university libraries and medical school libraries are helpful.
- For a small fee, you may also use computer data services such as Medline to seek out medical journal articles on the latest developments in your illness.

Finally, it's important for you *not* to feel stupid, intimidated, or fearful. Your doctor needs you to comply with the treatments she recommends, and that's best accomplished if you understand what she wants you to do and why. You have as much responsibility as your physician in your treatment.

GETTING A SECOND OPINION

Once you receive your diagnosis, you may experience some relief at finally having closure, yet you may not help but wonder if perhaps there might be another possibility. After all, your specialist was uncertain for so long, maybe she made a mistake. Or you might have found the specialist cold and blunt when she delivered the news. Perhaps you'd like to work with a doctor who expresses more warmth and compassion when dealing with you and your problems. Under any of these circumstances, you might decide that you would like an opinion from another physician. Indeed, it may be wise to obtain a second opinion, just to ease your mind.

But getting a second opinion is not as easy as it sounds. It feels so right and logical yet when you present the idea to your GP and ask for a referral to another specialist, he may seem almost displeased with you. This might confuse you. Doesn't your GP, like you, want to be sure that the diagnosis is correct? Doesn't he want you to work with a doctor with whom you feel comfortable? Why would he urge you to stay with the same specialist despite your expression of discontent?

There may be several reasons for this disinclination, and I believe knowing them will help you make your way through the sometimes confusing maze of modern medicine. To begin with, your GP might feel threatened by your questioning his judgment. Moreover, doctors often prefer working with colleagues whom they know and trust. Physicians usually maintain close working relationships with a number of specialists such as oncologists, cardiologists, neurologists, and surgeons, in networks that have developed over years of working together.

Doctors in a particular network keep frequent contact with one another, either informally on the telephone or formally at professional meetings. They may even see one another socially. These carefully developed relationships are important to your physician, emotionally and—to be frank—financially. They are important to you too, in your desire to get the best care possible.

Nevertheless, despite your general practitioner's biases, you are entitled to consult or seek treatment from whomever you wish. You must decide what is best for you.

Bear in mind that insurance companies willingly pay for second opinions; in some cases, especially when surgery is involved, they require them. You are bound to have a long relationship with the specialist you eventually choose to treat you, so why not feel comfortable and secure with that person from the start?

To get a new referral from your general practitioner, you must persuade him that it is essential to you psychologically to get a second opinion. You can say, for example, "I need to feel as secure with the specialist as I do with you." If your doctor still puts you off there are other alternatives:

- Ask friends, neighbors, or relatives about doctors with whom they have dealt.
- Ask friends, neighbors, or relatives if they know anyone who has had the disease and call that person for the name of their physician.
- Ask other medical personnel such as your dentist, urologist, or orthopedist. (These professionals get referrals from other physicians and usually know the community quite well.)
- Ask your state or county medical association for a list of board-certified specialists in your area.
- If there is a medical school in your community, inquire about specialists on the faculty. They are bound to be up on the latest research and some may have small private practices.
- Groups such as the American Diabetes Association, the National Multiple Sclerosis Society, or the American College of Obstetricians and Gynecologists provide referrals.

Some people are afraid of hurting the specialist's feelings when they seek a second opinion. It's important to handle this transition diplomatically. You might tell her that you want more information about your condition and so you are consulting with another specialist. You could say, for example, "I am extremely anxious and getting a second opinion would help calm me down." Rest assured that physicians are used to patients seeking outside confirmation, and some even encourage it.

You must also understand that getting a second opinion means just that—you are not discharging the first specialist. When you make your appointment with the new doctor, be clear with the receptionist that you are coming in for a *consultation.* You are not making a commitment to be the new specialist's patient just yet. This communicates to the second physician that you are gathering information and value an educated opinion.

After you've met with the consulting physician, you'll probably want to send him your X rays or other test results. You can obtain these from the first doctor's office by simply calling and requesting they be sent. Or you can hand-carry the records to the next appointment. These documents are yours, after all, and you are entitled to share them with the doctor rendering the second opinion.

The consultation can include additional tests, but when you have completed them, you may learn that the diagnosis is unchanged. At that point, you may decide that you like the manner of the first doctor better. Returning to her care, you have still benefitted from having a fresh pair of eyes look at your case.

If the diagnosis differs, however, it's important to seek a third, fourth, or even tenth opinion—do whatever you must. You'll want to reach a firm consensus. If several doctors agree on your diagnosis and treatment, you may feel more comfortable going ahead with the first physician's recommendations, say, for surgery. At the very least, you will have reassured yourself that you are pursuing the right course.

Sometimes, however, you may find that the consulting physician is reluctant to render his second opinion. That happened to me some years ago. I set up an appointment seeking a second opinion from a neurosurgeon after an orthopedist told me that I would need to wear a heavy back brace for the rest of my life because of a recurrent back problem.

The neurosurgeon examined me briefly. But then, rather than giving me another opinion or explaining why, he suggested that I return to my original orthopedic physician.

Instead of remaining quiet and feeling intimidated by this physician's reputation, I told him calmly, "Dr. Williams, if I hadn't wanted another opinion, I wouldn't have come to see you."

Dr. Williams walked out of the examining room. I felt stunned, hurt, and frustrated by what I perceived as a rejection. Alone in the examination room, I began to cry as I struggled to dress and replace the heavy brace. I heard a quiet knock on the door. It was Dr. Williams, asking to come in.

"I must apologize to you," he said. "I should never have avoided your questions. In fact, I believe you can discontinue the brace. You don't really need it anymore. You can use some exercises to strengthen your muscles."

Although Dr. Williams never told me why he didn't want to treat me, I guessed that he and my orthopedist were part of the same network. Perhaps he was reluctant to contradict an esteemed colleague. Doctors often protect each other in a sort of good-old-boy system, especially when it comes to dealing with patients. The lesson I learned here, however, was that had I not spoken up, I would still be wearing that cumbersome brace today. Not only did Dr. Williams offer me a second opinion, he also gave me hope and a new, less invasive treatment that ultimately helped heal my problem!

WHAT YOU SHOULD EXPECT FROM YOUR DOCTOR AND WHAT HE OR SHE SHOULD EXPECT FROM YOU

The moment you decide to remain under a specialist's care, you both have expectations about how to relate to each other. In order for the doctor-patient relationship to work well and to cement mutual trust, it's important to recognize that you are establishing an unwritten and unspoken contract with your physician. It may be unwritten for your doctor, but let me put it down on paper so these expectations are crystal clear:

WHAT YOUR DOCTOR EXPECTS OF YOU

1. You will follow her clear instructions.
2. You will accept what she tells you.
3. You will be considerate of her time.
4. You will give her important information.
5. You will be in charge of your situation.

WHAT YOU EXPECT OF YOUR DOCTOR

1. She will give you instructions.
2. She will give you the latest information.
3. She will respect your time.
4. She will listen to you.
5. She will allow you to make your own decisions.

You also have certain inalienable rights to determine what should be done with your body. These include:

1. The right to informed consent. Informed consent means that the procedure with all of its risks and benefits has been explained to you clearly so that you understand it, and once having understood, agree to it.

2. The right to choose treatment. You may reject a recommended treatment and ask for another. Can a doctor refuse to take care of you under these circumstances? If she feels you have not followed her instructions, frustrating her attempts to treat you, she can ask that you see someone else. But a doctor who fails to continue to provide care until you are accepted by another physician can be charged with abandonment and sued for malpractice.

Even in a hospital, you can decline X rays, laxatives, and excessive probing and puncturing of your body. Few have the courage to do so, since most patients act in ways they believe will please their doctors and nurses.

3. The right to see your records. The right of informed consent implies the right to know the truth. This may mean more than asking your doctor questions; it may require your seeing your medical records including X rays and lab reports. Doctors and hospitals have traditionally withheld these from patients, but in 1984, the American Medical Association advised that physicians make them available on patients' request.

4. The right to considerate care. This is the first item in the American Hospital Association's Patient's Bill of Rights published in 1973. There is no reason for you to accept inconsiderate and disrespectful treatment. Of course, you can't force a physician to behave properly, but if you're dissatisfied, you can speak up or seek alternative care.

5. The right to hospital treatment. Federal laws governing Medicare and Medicaid provide that any hospital participating in such programs must treat and accept medical emergencies, regardless of the patient's ability to pay.

6. The right to die. If you do not wish to be placed on a respirator or that heroic measures be taken to save your life, you must request that of your physician. She will not make this difficult decision for you.

You can and should break your unwritten contract with your physician (and look for a new doctor) if you:

- Are afraid to talk to her about your condition.
- Feel she has not given you the time and care you deserve.
- No longer trust her.
- Feel she has abandoned you.

Your doctor may forget, but you must never forget that you are paying her for expert advice. You can accept or reject that advice. After all, you are the one who is sick and anxious. She should be concerned with your feelings but you need not be worried about your doctor's to the same extent.

Since you have a chronic illness and your association with your doctor will most likely continue for many years, it's best to establish the boundaries of your relationship from the beginning. It's up to you to make your expectations clear. Let her know how you want her to treat you. Tell her that you'd appreciate it if she responds to your phone calls promptly, because you get anxious if she doesn't, or that you would prefer to see her, and not an assistant or nurse, when you come in for your monthly checkup.

It's also helpful to apprise your physician of your style. Some patients would rather not know all the gory details of their illness. Others crave information. However you choose to deal with the situation, put your physician on notice. If hearing the whole story makes you too anxious, let your specialist know in advance. If, on the other hand, you're a question-asker like I am, tell the doctor that you'll be querying her about your condition or why she has prescribed certain medications and treatments. You might say "I need answers to help me feel less frightened."

You must also remember that your doctor and her staff are human and fallible. They will make mistakes. Nevertheless, if there's anything about your physician's treatment that you find disagreeable, you should be able to discuss it. This includes being kept waiting for a long time or dealing with an impolite staff member. Most physicians are blameless in this regard, but if yours is not, you should make her aware of your feelings. Rudeness notwithstanding, you should remember that this behavior in no way reflects your doctor's ability to treat you. It may simply indicate a lack of concern for the way her office is run.

How should you approach your physician if you feel mistreated? Suppose you are angry and frustrated because she has kept you waiting for two hours. Keep calm and deal with the situation diplomatically. Before or after your examination, you might say "I did my best to get here on time, but then I spent two hours in the waiting room. I appreciate that you have emergencies but you must understand that I have missed two hours of work. Perhaps next time your staff can call me to reschedule if you're going to be so late." Of course if the delay is unconscionably long and your physician's attitude unapologetic, you may wish to seek out a physician who will be more respectful and responsive.

You should also expect that your physician, and not an associate, will perform an agreed upon procedure. If you're scheduled for surgery, be sure that her name appears on the release form. This is your life, after all, and you want to be in charge of it.

THE DOCTOR'S DILEMMA

After the initial diagnosis, you may meet with your specialist many times over a period of months or years, perhaps even for the rest of your life. She may take charge of your case, acting as "quarterback" for the rest of your medical team. You may even find that despite this deep involvement, over time your specialist or even your GP seems to become less responsive to your case.

To understand how this can occur, it's best to recognize why people are attracted to the practice of medicine in the first place. Often prospective physicians apply to medical school because they have witnessed family members suffering from intractable diseases. They enter the profession with a profound desire to cure illnesses. Their training reinforces the urge to heal: they are taught to do whatever possible to sustain life. Consequently, they derive deep gratification from being able to restore their patients to health.

Yet a chronic illness may frustrate a physician's basic desires and training. It may be extremely difficult for a doctor to pronounce a diagnosis of chronic illness, especially if she identifies with you in some way. (She may, for instance, relate your case to her own situation or to that of her spouse, child, or parent.) Moreover, if your physician has little to offer you in the way of treatment, she and her staff may lose interest—not in *you* but in *your case*. She has been trained to heal, not to sit on her hands!

In order for this relationship to remain productive, you must be realistic. Your physician and medical science may be limited in how much they can help you. But you are entitled to your feelings. If you believe that you are getting short shrift, communicate openly with your doctor and express your feelings. If you do this in a nonthreatening manner, you will find that she'll probably respond empathetically. For example, you could say "I recognize that you may be frustrated with my condition, but I need more of your attention. I feel uncared for."

Doctors and their staffs recognize that they get burned out in their work. But until you point it out in a way that they can hear, they may not realize how they have presented themselves on a given day. Your speaking up will spare you feelings of resentment and will help to keep the relationship on an even keel.

HOW TO AVOID FEELING
VICTIMIZED BY THE PROCESS

Although I made the point earlier that you should not underestimate the importance of your relationship to your physicians, it's also crucial that you not overestimate it. Since you may be feeling weak and vulnerable at this time, you may become overly dependent on your medical caretakers and may surrender to them too much power. Indeed, you may become so fearful of upsetting your doctor or his staff that you accept behavior that under other circumstances you would find objectionable.

This is what happened to Michelle, a forty-year-old boutique manager. As she sat in my office, pouring out her story, I recognized that her experience didn't reflect that of most patients. Yet sadly such situations occur often enough that they leave a good many people in a state of confusion and despair.

"Last week, I had my first visit with the specialist whom my general practitioner recommended," Michelle reported, wringing a damp tissue in her hands. "I was afraid that something was terribly wrong with me, but I had no idea what it was. I was really petrified.

"I sat in the waiting room for over an hour for an appointment I had made a month ago. When the nurse finally called me into an examining room, she handed me a sheet and told me to get undressed. I spent another thirty minutes nearly naked, sitting on one of those tables. I swear, for a full half hour I was shivering from fear and cold!

"When the doctor finally came in, he didn't apologize for being so late. In fact, he hardly introduced himself at all. He just rushed through his examination. Afterward, he listened to my medical history, but he never even looked up at me. While I was talking to him, he took a few phone calls from other doctors (and one from his stockbroker too) and went through his mail.

"Just when I felt ready to ask all the questions I had been preparing for days, he stood up and was on his way out the door. I felt so alone and scared. While I was getting dressed, I decided to call him once I got home, but then I hesitated. He seemed so busy and important, I just hated to bother him. I was also afraid that he would think I was a hypochondriac or a hysterical female. Besides, he doesn't know what's wrong with me yet. He didn't give me a diagnosis. He just suggested a few possibilities, but nothing definite.

"Irene," Michelle continued, "there were so many questions I wanted to ask. Now I'm torn about what to do. I'm used to talking to my GP. Shouldn't I feel comfortable talking to the specialist too? After all, my GP recommended him."

I explained to Michelle that she probably felt uncomfortable for several reasons: This was her first meeting with this doctor. He knew very little about her condition and certainly less about her personally. I supported her in her perception that he had treated her in a dismissive and brusque manner.

Then I said, "You know, Michelle, normally in your everyday life and work, you're an assertive person; you wouldn't let anyone push you around like that. My hunch is that you feel vulnerable and frightened about your symptoms. Maybe that has weakened your will for the moment. I'm sure your instincts are correct but you're afraid to follow them."

I advised her to speak up during subsequent appointments. I said, "Michelle, maybe Dr. Jones was preoccupied. You might want to give him another chance and try to get his attention. Why don't you say 'Dr. Jones, you came highly recommended. I was very upset last week when I had to wait. Then you seemed to be in a hurry—too busy for me to ask questions. But I do need you to hear them and respond.'

"If he responds, 'Gee, I'm sorry I kept you waiting. Go ahead. I'll try to answer your questions,' you may feel less victimized. But if, after speaking up, you still feel that he's giving you inadequate attention, you can either learn to live with his personality or change doctors. You do have a choice."

DEVELOPING A PARTNERSHIP
WITH YOUR DOCTOR'S STAFF

As you embark upon your relationship with your chosen specialist, it's important to realize that you're beginning an association with members of her staff too, including her receptionist, office and financial managers, office nurses and assistants, and hospital nurses.

During the course of your treatment, you'll be dealing with several (if not many) nurses. They can advise and inform the doctor but they must follow her orders explicitly; these take precedence over all others. Besides, the doctor or the hospital hires and pays the nurses, so there are financial reasons for them to follow orders.

Particularly during hospitalization, you will be spending more time with the nursing staff than with the doctor. The hospital nurses will be your physician's surrogates while you are under her care. Indeed, the nurses are the people with whom you and your family will interact the most. You will be developing an intense association with them, one that usually begins under trying circumstances.

Your relationship to your nurses will differ from what you've developed with your physician. In fact, you're likely to have a more intimate physical and emotional connection with your hospital nurses than with your doctor. They will touch you, sometimes causing pain (when they give you an injection), and sometimes soothingly (when they rub you down or shampoo you). They may witness you crying or screaming and will overhear your conversations as you talk on the phone or with visitors. They may note everything you and your family do or say on your chart—even how you behave with them. Sometimes they will be the "unwelcome messenger" of ill tidings.

However, although the nurses may know you more intimately than your doctor, they may have less ability to respond to your appeals. You may feel disappointed in their reluctance to fulfill your expressed needs. Nevertheless, they are duty bound to follow doctor's orders, even if that means waiting three hours to change your medication because your physician is still in surgery.

Your hospital nurses are part of a team. They alternate shifts with one another and share responsibility for your care. The outgoing nursing staff must communicate your progress to the incoming shift. The nurses in your physician's office, on the other hand, are not part of a rotating team. They have more access to your doctor and may be more available to answer your questions than she is.

As with the physicians who are treating you, you also have an unwritten contract with the nursing staff. However, this relationship is more ambiguous because, for the most part, the nurses are not calling the shots—they are simply following your doctor's instructions. Thus, nurses may find themselves in a double bind: they are not fully in authority, yet they are left in charge of your care.

WHAT YOUR NURSES EXPECT OF YOU	WHAT YOU EXPECT OF YOUR NURSES
1. You will *cooperate* with them.	1. The doctor has given them the right orders.
2. You will *comply* with their treatment.	2. They know what they're doing.
3. You will *inform* them of how you feel.	3. They will respond to your needs and get help.
4. You will be *reasonable* in your demands.	4. They will respond reasonably to your requests.
5. You will be more passive with them than with the doctor.	5. They will allow you to be more dependent.
6. You will caution your family about being overly intrusive.	6. They will respect your family's requests.

THE NURSING STAFF AND YOUR FAMILY

The potential for clashes between nurses and family members is high. Many nurses feel (and rightly so) that they have authority and responsibility for your hospital care. It is often difficult for family members to let go. Your loved ones may rail at the fact that your nurse didn't bring your medication on time or freshen your bed clothing. If they feel out of control, giving the nurses orders may make them feel as if they're helping you. Besides, your family doesn't want to be left out of the decision-making process. Their involvement with your treatment gives them something tangible to do.

Consequently, your family may experience the nurse's hostility for getting in her way and looking over her shoulder. While the physician may chat with your family for a few minutes and leave, the nurses will see your family whenever they walk into your room. They may feel the family's intrusion into their territory and may battle for control over it.

Most good nurses understand that caretaking family members often know more than they do about the patient's emotional needs. They not only cooperate with family members but respect them and seek their help in feeding and cheering the patient. You must understand their role and their feelings about it, but mostly you must understand your rights and expectations as a hospital patient and exert them.

Unfortunately, the nurses caring for my infant son were unwilling to take into consideration my knowledge of my son's condition, and I was afraid to assert myself. Until I had to face my children's serious, life-threatening illnesses, all of my interactions with doctors and nurses had been positive. These were people, after all, who cared about me and responded to me when I needed them. They cured me. My first exposure to a different kind of treatment shattered all of my previous expectations.

Our third child, Kenneth Jay, was born with a serious assortment of heart defects. When he was about seven months old, our son became so desperately ill that my pediatrician suggested I take him immediately to Baltimore, an hour from my home, where he was under the general care of a famous children's heart specialist. Thus, in the middle of a hot summer day, I made a tearful call to my husband and set out from Washington, D.C., grabbing diapers, bottles, and whatever I thought I'd need. I had no idea how long we would stay.

Upon arriving, I settled into the small hospital room feeling relieved that I had brought my baby to a "safe" place where he would receive expert care if a problem arose. This was not to be the case.

At home, I had become accustomed to Jay-Jay's breathing difficulties and would feed him whenever he could suck. All I had to do was go to the refrigerator and retrieve his bottle. In the hospital, however, the nurses would not allow me to keep anything in his room, including a bottle warmer. I would have to ask them for the heated bottles. Rules were rules.

Unfortunately, Jay-Jay knew and cared nothing about hospital protocol. He could not suppress his needs until I summoned a nurse, waited for her to come, gave her my request, and received the warmed bottle some thirty or more minutes later. Consequently, when he became hungry and I could not satisfy him, he began crying frantically. This, of course, weakened him still further.

Explaining this dilemma to the nurses made no difference to them. Indeed, when I asked for a bottle that evening and waited for over an hour, holding my wailing, panicky baby in my arms, I became so desperate that I literally ran out of the room, down two flights of stairs to the exit, and out onto the streets of downtown Baltimore. My vague notion was to go home. However, after a few minutes, I realized that I had forgotten my handbag in the hospital room. I sheepishly returned, but never told anyone of my experience.

What should I have done under the circumstances? I was young (in my twenties) and inexperienced. I didn't understand the chain of command or know who to turn to for help. I felt intimidated by the nurses' authoritarian manner. If this situation had occurred today, I would have confronted the nurses more forcefully about the problem. If they were still intransigent, I would have approached their supervisor or the head nurse. Failing that, I would have called the cardiologist. She would have instructed the nurses to allow me to feed my baby on demand, since it was in his best interest to do so. Without doctor's orders, however, the nurses were powerless to act on his behalf.

You can confront the nursing staff with your specific problems. Be firm and clear about what you need without being a pain in the neck and without raising your voice. You could say, for example, "I understand the rules and I respect you. But this situation is causing my sick baby to be even sicker. I understand your position. Who do I call to help me?"

Some people hesitate to confront a nurse about her behavior, fearing that somehow she has the power to harm them if they express dissatisfaction. Rest assured that nurses are professionals. No matter how they feel about you or your family personally, they would never undermine your care. They can, however, increase your stress in an already stressful situation. It's up to you to recognize their human frailties, but also to make sure that your needs are met.

FINDING THE RIGHT DOCTOR

The best way to ensure a good doctor-patient relationship is to invest the time to find the right match from the start. Certainly, training, board certification, and experience with a certain procedure or disease are all important aspects of finding the right doctor. But I believe that much of the doctor-patient relationship is purely subjective. If you and she don't hit it off, then she won't be right for you, no matter what her other qualifications. In order to find the right match you must feel that:

- You trust your doctor's judgment.
- She cares about you.
- She will be responsive to you.

This is the ideal, and it is possible to achieve. The Clarks, another family I had worked with, were able to locate two doctors with whom they had developed an excellent rapport. The general practitioner, neurologist, and I collaborated in a real team effort on this case, even though none of us shared the same office space. The Clarks reaped the benefits: they never had to complain, they got answers to all of their questions, and they felt safe and well cared for. That's the ultimate goal of forging an effective doctor-patient relationship.

REMEMBER

- It's your life and you are paying for advice and services.
- Your doctor and her staff are human and fallible.
- Unless you are informed, you cannot be responsible and in control of your medical decisions.
- It may be wise—or even necessary—to get a second opinion.
- Be as realistic as possible regarding your relationship to your physician. Make sure that you feel comfortable with her. It can affect how you respond to her treatments.
- Don't allow yourself to be intimidated. Always inform your physician when you are unhappy with any aspect of your treatment. A good doctor will not feel threatened.

THINGS TO DO

- Seek a second opinion if you're dissatisfied with the specialist or feel uncertain about the diagnosis.
- Get as much information about your disease as is possible, but only as much as you're comfortable with. It should help with your treatment.
- If you are anxious in your doctor's office, bring in prepared questions and take notes. Have someone accompany you.
- Share your feelings and concerns with your doctor and her staff, especially if you feel you're being mistreated.
- If you're going into surgery, put your surgeon's name on the release form. This will insure that she will be performing the operation and not another member of the medical team.
- Get copies of your medical records if it helps you to keep track of your treatment.
- Speak up clearly if you're dissatisfied with a nurse's treatment of you. Start by speaking with her directly. If that doesn't work, speak to the head nurse, and then with your doctor.

Part II

TAKING
CHARGE

5.

Mastering Your Fear of Loss of Control

===

Ever since your diagnosis and perhaps for the first time in your life, you must make decisions based on a present you can't control and a future you can't predict. These decisions may be relatively insignificant or they may have far-reaching consequences, from determining how to shower in the morning when you can no longer depend on your legs to hold you up to evaluating if you should marry and have children when you're unsure if your diabetes will cause you to end up in a wheelchair.

You may have to factor in physical and psychological considerations. For example, you may be wondering what to do about an arm that constantly swells or how to contain the anger you feel toward your healthy spouse. You may also need to make practical adjustments, such as having to move into a ground-floor apartment because you can no longer manage stairs.

Your disability may advance so slowly (as in the case of some cancers, cardiovascular disease, and multiple sclerosis) that at times you may even forget that you were ever diagnosed. On the other hand, your affliction may strike rapidly and without warning (as in the case of a heart attack or stroke). But however your ailment progresses, you may be unable to control flare-ups and recurrences.

It may seem to you as if your illness (and not you) is in control of your life. Indeed, you may find that your disease has begun to dominate and dictate your every move. It is a force to be reckoned with, and its unpredictability may be its most powerful element. You fear that you are losing control.

THE CONSEQUENCES OF LOSS OF CONTROL

What happens when you perceive you're no longer master of your destiny? Under these circumstances, most people feel disoriented. This is a normal and expectable response. Indeed, you may sense that your general frame of reference has changed—that all of your old anchors are gone. Traits you could count on, such as high energy or quick reflexes, may no longer be available to you.

All of your usual coping mechanisms may be challenged. If jogging three miles a day was your favorite way to alleviate stress, you may feel deprived of that escape valve now that your heart is weak. Or you may have taken great pleasure in going out to dinner and a movie every Saturday night, but now shun restaurants and theaters because of your difficulty maneuvering a wheelchair in a crowd.

Moreover, your view of the world may have changed. You may have once seen it as compassionate and sympathetic, but now it feels hard and cruel. You may run into the problem Donald did. For ten years, he felt lucky to work under a boss who was generous and supportive. But once Donald contracted AIDS, he could no longer put in the ten-hour workdays his supervisor required. This same boss now acted uncaringly and unsupportively toward him.

Indeed, your universe may have always turned in one direction, but now it may feel as if it has suddenly stopped in midcourse and reversed itself. You may find that just as you were reaching your prime money-making years, you can no longer be productive in your career. Or, like Brian, a young man who came to see me after being diagnosed with Hodgkin's disease, you may have to let go of your hard-fought independence and move back with your parents because you can no longer take care of yourself.

These situations may leave you emotionally vulnerable. Feeling frightened and different, your self-confidence may have been shattered. You may wonder if others will still love and respect you in your new condition. You may perceive yourself as inadequate. Even a small incident, such as dropping your wallet because your hands are trembling due to Parkinson's disease, may make you feel naked and exposed. And you may feel shame, as another patient did when she heard strange sounds coming out of her mouth as a result of her stroke.

THE PSYCHOLOGICAL TUG-OF-WAR

Your illness is a physical problem, but you are struggling with its emotional effects daily. You believe that you and your disease are engaged in a psychological tug-of-war, and right now your illness has the upper hand.

That power struggle may have begun even before your official diagnosis, during that seemingly interminable period in which you were waiting for your physician to give a formal name to your collection of symptoms. During this extremely anxious interval, some people will reach for any control they can find. Loretta, for example, told me she would take any diagnosis, even cancer, just to be alleviated of the unbearable agony of not knowing. People like Loretta believe that once they have identified the illness, they can do something about it. Unfortunately, they don't realize that even if they have the diagnosis in hand, they may still be powerless to change their medical situation.

The truth is, many chronic illnesses offer little in the way of treatment, or the available treatment may not ensure a cure. This may sound bleak, but remember, *even if you cannot control your body, you can still control your mind.* You are in charge of your responses to your disease. You have this power no matter what your disease dictates, so you do retain ultimate control over your life.

Recent research in the new field of psychoneuro-immunology suggests that the mind not only can control your life, but it can also control the course of your disease. In one important investigation to which I alluded earlier, Dr. David Spiegel of Stanford University Medical School studied women with advanced breast cancer. He wanted to know if those who were enrolled in a counseling support group fared better than those who were not. His findings, published in 1989 in the prestigious British medical journal *The Lancet,* indicated that the women who received counseling lived twice as long since the study began as those who had received only medical care without counseling.

The message here is that your emotional state can affect your physical condition, your symptoms, and even the progression of your illness. No physical ailment can wrest complete control away from you. Even if you think that you are helpless in face of your disorder and that your fate is in the hands of others such as your doctors or God, you are still the master. Even if you can no longer direct how you live physically, you can always maintain power over how you live psychologically.

To demonstrate just how influential the mind can be over the body, I sometimes ask my patients to participate in a little exercise. I first tell them of my intense fear of being suspended in space—I'm terrified of sitting in a cable car, for example, dangling between two mountaintops. Then, while I'm imagining this terrifying scenario, I ask them to place a hand on my pulse. They inevitably note my sweaty, shaking hands. The act of creating that mental image, even while safe in my office, brings this reaction on and makes my heart pound.

However, since this is only an abstract product of my imagination, I can also make the image and my reaction to it disappear. I understand that I have not been dangling in a cable car—this was not a real event. My stress diminishes when I realize that I know what caused my sweaty hands and pounding heart; if I stop thinking about the cable car, my distress will go away.

It seems strange to discover that a fear can affect your body so forcefully. Even if your rational self knows that you are in no danger, your body may continue to respond to irrational thoughts. But the mind is a powerful tool. Just as it can conjure negative feelings, so can it produce *positive energy*. Overcoming your fear of loss of control can add to that positive energy. Throughout the rest of this chapter, I'll be giving you advice on just how to do that.

CONTROL: HANGING ON, LETTING GO, LOSING IT

How you come to terms with your loss of control is a purely individual matter. I have found that some individuals maintain control, no matter what the consequences, while others become quite passive; still others simply lose control and come unglued temporarily. Indeed, all three reactions are normal. You could experience any one of them and maybe even several at different stages in your disease. Just bear in mind that they are temporary reactions to your new situation. Let's look at these three coping styles more closely.

Hanging On

People who feel the need to exert immediate control may move swiftly to make major life decisions. They can move too quickly, reacting before the full scope of their disease has been ascertained. In his haste to do "something, anything," Kenneth left a successful career as a stockbroker, only to discover subsequently that his disease had been misdiagnosed. Too late, he learned that he could have avoided a major family upheaval had he waited for confirmation.

Audrey gave up her corporate job and decided to move back to her home town to be with her grandparents within hours of her diagnosis of multiple sclerosis. Although it would take years before her disease would progress to the stage that it incapacitated her, she felt it necessary to cut all her ties to her current life in an attempt to regain control.

Others with the same powerful need to exert control may undertake unproven treatments, bizarre diets, or unauthorized medication.

Letting Go

Other individuals become utterly passive in the face of their diagnosis. They want others to take care of them, to make their medical decisions for them, to change their lifestyles for them.

Charlene, a bright, well-educated, capable woman followed that route. After being diagnosed with Parkinson's, she retreated from life, demanding that her family take complete charge. She carried her passivity to such a point that she even allowed her husband to choose books for her at the library. She had given up all sense of self-respect and in her family's eyes had become a "nothing." She was unaware of how passively she was behaving until her husband and daughter expressed their resentment.

In working with Charlene, I pointed out to her that she could accomplish some tasks on her own. She was capable of performing certain household chores, answering the phone, and cooking. After realizing that she was taking advantage of her family's good nature, she took more control of her life.

Sometimes, however, seemingly passive individuals will convince themselves and others that they have given up control of their lives, when in truth they are still directing the decision-making process. That was the case with Marta, a fifty-two-year-old woman in a state of depression who came to see me.

Two weeks after her husband had died, Marta was diagnosed with cervical cancer. She was frightened for her future, and understandably so, having received two such enormous blows one after the other. But as she put it, she "allowed" her two daughters Janet and Lucy, to "convince" her that the upkeep of her house would now be too much for her. So, soon after her diagnosis, Marta packed up her belongings and her two cats and moved from her cozy little home in a small town to an apartment in a big city where both daughters lived. She decided that her older daughter, Janet, should be responsible for her care.

It was Janet who made the appointment for Marta to see me. She even brought her mother in, although Marta lived within walking distance. At first it appeared to me that Marta had surrendered control over her life to her daughters. As she spoke, however, she revealed her anger toward them, Janet in particular. "She promised me so much," Marta complained, "but she really isn't there for me. The only reason I made this big move is that I expected Janet to take care of me. I thought she'd watch over my health and take me out shopping and to the movies."

"Well, how often does she contact you?" I asked.

"She calls every day, but she brings me over to her house for dinner only once a week. I know she's busy with her work and her own family. She's been having some trouble with her husband lately, and one of her children is recuperating from a car accident, but I'm really lonely here. I miss my old life and my good friends and neighbors. I miss the smallness and familiarity of my hometown. I'm really sorry I let my daughters take over my life. They made me do things I would have never done on my own."

Listening to this woman's complaints, I felt it imperative that Marta understand that she, and not her daughters, had made the decision to move. So I said, "Marta, although it seems to you as if you've turned control of your life over to your daughters, you're still the one making the decisions. You may be unhappy with your situation today, but you need to understand that you made your choice under duress. Given your state of vulnerability, it was natural for you to want someone to take over and look after you. It was probably easy to misread your daughter's generous offer. My hunch is that you were feeling needy and that you imagined Janet and her family could fill the gap left by your husband."

Marta and I spent several hours contemplating her present dilemma and how she could make some peace with herself. Ultimately, after reviewing her options, Marta once more acknowledged her autonomy. She decided that she still wanted to live in the same city as her daughters, but that she would feel more comfortable with her younger child, Lucy. Now, Marta had a clearer picture of what she could and could not expect her children to do for her.

While Charlene was an essentially passive person, content with her lot in life until her family complained, Marta was passive only for the moment. She really did have her own desires, thoughts, and goals. And once she got back in touch with them, she was once more able to make her own decisions and stand by them.

Losing It

Some people with a strong need for control simply lose it when faced with a medical crisis. They then often go through a "crazy" period, during which their emotions seem to run wild before they regain a sense of stability. Under these circumstances, it helps them to remember that these feelings are temporary.

Dorothy learned this the hard way, a few months after her firstborn child was diagnosed with cystic fibrosis. Dorothy simply couldn't handle the news. She became irrational, fantasizing that her infant would disappear so that she could have a healthy one. Even her parents went a little "nuts," suggesting that she leave her husband and baby, so much did they want Dorothy's life to return to "normal." Fortunately, however, her older sister was sensitive enough to recognize her sister's agitated state and brought her in to see me.

Given Dorothy's history, I could easily empathize. She had married late and was eager to have children before her biological clock ran out. However, to complicate matters, at the time of the baby's diagnosis, Dorothy's husband, Jim, was up for an important job in another country. Dorothy feared that the foreign country could not offer adequate medical care for their son in case of an emergency. Her sister was a physician, so she understood this need well. She did not want to make the move from her cozy Virginia town, but more important, she didn't want to deal with her sick baby.

HOW TO REGAIN CONTROL

Dorothy struggled to regain control of her life and her feelings, especially since she was so undone by the bad news. Together, we gradually unraveled her problems, dealing with them one at a time. Ordinarily stable individuals, when faced with deep stress, can forget their basic coping skills. Although Dorothy and her family were all solid people, they felt overwhelmed by their need to deal with all their intersecting problems at once. I helped them to revert to their usual commonsense thinking and find solutions for each of their problems individually.

I did so, by helping them (and my other patients) to:

- Separate the immediate problems from the long-term ones.
- Make their own decisions wherever possible (especially regarding medical needs) and do what they can do about the illness.
- Evaluate and change what's changeable.
- Pinpoint areas of stress.
- Set reachable and reasonable goals that help reduce stress.
- Salvage what they can of old coping mechanisms.
- Use stress reduction techniques.
- Evaluate to whom they can turn when the going gets rough.
- Be flexible and creative.
- Join support groups.
- Plan ahead.
- Use the power of the mind.

Let's look at these coping skills more closely, for I believe they can help you, too, regain a sense of control in your life.

Separating the Long Term from the Short Term

Chronic illnesses rarely strike when there's nothing else going on in your life. Most often, they overlay other problems that exist in the family. Believing that you have to resolve all your problems at once, as did Dorothy, may leave you feeling overwhelmed. In order to take charge, it's important to sort out the issues and decide which problems are immediate and which are long-term. You can then prioritize how you cope with them. You could choose to dispense with the immediate problems first, or you may feel more comfortable resolving the long-term issues.

I helped Dorothy and her family separate their child's illness from the decision to take a job promotion in another country. After all, they couldn't do much about their child's condition (the long-term problem), but they did have some leeway in deciding where Jim would work and where they would live (the short-term problem). I asked Dorothy and Jim to consider what they would have done if their child were well. Then I had them factor in the new elements (the diagnosis and its ramifications). In this way, the couple was able to think clearly again, eliminating the anxiety that the diagnosis had prompted.

It might be wise for you to list your problems. You might note alternative solutions next to each issue. Of course, while some obstacles remain insurmountable or there may be little you can do about them, you may find solutions to other issues that you previously thought were insoluble.

Make Your Own Decisions

Neither how you make decisions nor the decisions you actually make are as important as the fact that you are the person doing the deciding. That's the essence of taking charge.

Making their own decisions helped Marta and Dorothy reexperience the feeling of being in control. Marta decided to look to her younger daughter for support. It took Dorothy several weeks, but finally she regained her equilibrium by realizing that she was a grown woman capable of choices. On her own, she opted to remain with her husband and baby. After researching the medical facilities in the foreign country, she decided that she could go along with Jim's taking this important new job.

Your choices are idiosyncratic. In fact, they may seem downright odd to someone else, but doing things your way is vitally important in your attempt to regain control of your life. One woman in my practice, Thelma, had always enjoyed testing others' reactions to her by being outrageous. "By golly," she proclaimed in my office one day, "cancer isn't going to stop me from being me!" To the world, her way of controlling her environment challenged understanding: having gone bald from chemotherapy, this woman attended black-tie affairs without wearing any head covering. But for Thelma the experience was therapeutic, because she hadn't backed down from her usual stance in the world.

MEDICAL DECISIONS

It may be frightening to take responsibility for your own medical decisions. Many individuals give up all control to their doctors—they refuse to participate in their own care. But by becoming more involved, you can help regain a sense of control over your disease.

Take Stephanie, who was diagnosed with breast cancer at the age of forty-four. Her tumor was relatively small and her lymph nodes were uninvolved, so she underwent a lumpectomy and radiation. However, because of her age, there was a small chance that the cancer could return—the recurrence rate for a person in her situation was about 7 percent.

Stephanie's oncologist had offered her the option of chemotherapy in addition to surgery and radiation. "It will shave another 2 percent off the recurrence rate," he explained.

Although Stephanie was neither required to undergo chemo nor eager to do so, she opted for the more aggressive course, especially since her father had died of cancer less than two years earlier. At the end of her treatment, she felt that she had done everything she could to lick the disease. She had successfully participated with her physician in making a medical decision and felt good about taking charge of her life once more.

Evaluate and Change What Is Changeable

To take control, it's also important for you to look at your life before your illness and then consider how the disease has affected it. In that way you will separate the hard realities of your "old" life from the abstractions of your illness. Your thinking should take the following progression:

1. Consider what was important to you prior to your illness.
2. Evaluate how that may or may not have changed since your diagnosis.
3. What part or parts of your old life can remain intact?
4. Where will you need to make changes?

Your evaluation will be based on the premise that rather than losing all that is meaningful in your life, with a bit of creative thinking, you can preserve much of what you have always valued. Once you allow yourself to look at painful feelings, you have the power to move away from them at will.

Tom was a seriously ill young man when I first met him and his wife, Sally. In fact, the day before their first appointment with me, Tom's doctors had informed him that he had only six months to live. He had been diagnosed with lupus erythematosus some ten years earlier; over the years he had experienced a number of flares, but the illness had always been manageable with bed rest and good care. Now, however, doctors warned that any new flare-up could be his last. His kidneys were close to failure, a situation that was beyond Tom and Sally's control.

When I saw this couple, they were desperately, tearfully trying to hold on to some measure of control, even while they felt helpless and hopeless. Wisely, Sally, a psychologist, sought professional help in anticipation of the difficult times ahead.

Several days after our first meeting, Sally called with exciting news. Tom's condition was less severe than originally suspected. He did have a chance to live, but he would have to make drastic changes in his diet and life-style. Recognizing the difficulty in complying, Sally asked me to help them adjust.

We began by looking at what Tom needed to change immediately. Obviously, the simplest was his diet, which presented a pleasant challenge since Tom loved to cook.

The second step was more difficult. Tom had been the major breadwinner in the family, but now he needed to curtail the scope of his work. Tom's career as an economist had involved a great deal of traveling. In his present condition, he was incapable of negotiating airports and long international flights. He was deeply saddened by this loss because he loved his work. "Where will I find the same kind of gratification that my career gives me?" he wondered. He was at his peak and feared that he would now have to give it all up.

As we continued this difficult and often painfully realistic evaluation of the changes Tom needed to make, we discovered that all was not lost. Tom realized that he had developed enough of a reputation as a fine economist to become a home-based private consultant. We compiled a list of companies and agencies that might wish to hire him.

Sally, a highly skilled clinician, had returned to part-time work after the birth of their son four years earlier. Until the current crisis, she had regarded her career as a pleasurable outside activity. Now Sally was able to step in to make up the shortfall in family income. She offered to work full-time. She said, "Look, Tom, if you can handle Joshua when he comes home from preschool and do the cooking, I'll manage a full-time practice." As a result of our analyzing where change was possible, this family was able to adjust to the vicissitudes of Tom's disease.

Pinpoint Areas of Stress

By identifying which parts of your life are stressful, you can more clearly see what you can do about changing them. If, for example, your job or coworkers create a lot of negativity in your life, you might consider working for a new company or transferring to a different department. If you can't arrange this, try altering your schedule or reducing your hours. If you're having trouble managing steep steps or a long walk from the parking lot to your office, you might need to arrange another way to get to work—for instance, carpooling with a coworker who could drop you off at the main entrance.

One of my patients, Janice, described the personal torture she endured daily from Sharon, the woman whose desk faced hers. Janice suffered from Sharon's constant, unrelenting stream of chatter, but because she didn't want to hurt Sharon's feelings, she never voiced her complaints. Soon, however, Janice began feeling depressed: she was trapped between her desire to keep her good job and her inability to make her need for peace and quiet known. Once we had pinpointed this area of stress, Janice was able to plan a way to ask her colleague to curb the monologue.

In my office she rehearsed what she would say: "Sharon, I don't know if you're aware that you talk to me constantly. Since I've gotten sick, my nerves aren't as good as they used to be. My doctor says I need more quiet. I like you and I'm interested in what you're doing. But right now, I need more quiet at my desk. I hope you don't mind. Let's have lunch and we can talk as much as we want."

Set Reachable Goals over Which You Can Have Control

When I was highly stressed after my daughter Linda's first surgery at the age of four, I began gardening with a vengeance. Every day, I sprayed my roses at 8 A.M. and thinned the tomato plants at ten—a ritual I never broke. I didn't know why I was doing it, only that it made me feel better. Gardening was my way of dealing with days filled with the terror that my daughter's delicate heart surgery would fail. These simple tasks provided me with quick, satisfying resolutions and instant gratification. For the moment, I was master of my environment.

Of course, gardening didn't solve my big problems. But it did give me a badly needed respite: time to feel in control of the world around me and to get results that I could see, touch, and even enjoy.

Think about activities in which you could engage to achieve the same results. You might take a fifteen-minute walk around the block, wash your hair, clean a closet, knit another twenty-five rows, sew buttons on your son's baseball shirt, paint a room, or wax the car. You've set a reachable goal and accomplished it!

Sometimes maintaining rituals such as these helps to make you feel more in control. You might wish to attend religious services regularly or cook dinner every night. One patient insisted on arranging her grown daughter's birthday party, even though she had come home from the hospital after triple bypass surgery less than two weeks earlier. She had always given the party in the past and didn't want her surgery to interfere. So she maintained the family ritual, taking short rests every ten minutes, as her body dictated.

These stabilizing rituals may even take a strange form in someone else's eyes. Felicia sat in her dying husband's hospital room, directly across from his bed, applying and reapplying fresh nail polish to her long fingernails. This was her way of maintaining equilibrium.

Salvage What You Can of Old Coping Mechanisms

How have your defenses worked for you in the past? Can you use them now? Consider whether some of your old coping mechanisms are still available. Try to be realistic if they're not. For example, some people ward off depression by performing a strenuous physical activity such as running while others busy themselves with myriad activities to avoid thinking about their problems. If you find that your disease no longer allows you to run, you might consider other, related activities such as "running" an organization from your home. In this way, you can salvage from the activity what you had always enjoyed.

I had one patient who took this advice literally. Completely immobilized by his advanced amyotrophic lateral sclerosis (a fast-moving, devastating, incurable disease that destroys the muscles' ability to move), Jeffrey sponsored a running benefit to raise funds for his local chapter of the ALS society. Another young man dying of AIDS who had been a successful stage manager managed the fund-raising and building of a state-of-the-art special-care AIDS clinic that would bear his name.

It helps to have an activity to look forward to even if, in the larger scheme of things, it seems insignificant. The anticipation projects you into the future and away from today's unhappiness. Even if you have planned ahead for an event that you cannot physically accomplish by the appointed date, you'll still have derived some pleasure from the prospect of a future enjoyment. Think of it as giving yourself a gift when you're feeling down.

Also consider this idea as a possibility: even while you feel as if you are falling apart, you may not be; this may just be the way you're coping. If your behavior seems uncharacteristic or excessive—crying incessantly, talking inordinately, or even avoiding human contact—this may be what you need to do for the moment in order to recoup. If it helps you get through the night, then so be it.

Dorothy needed to fantasize her lost "perfect" baby until she realized how "crazy" that was. Sally was near hysteria by the time she came into my office. Yet both women were able to reassert control of their lives after taking the time to ponder their options. Several years ago, when I was going through a difficult period and thought I was falling apart, I came across a billboard that read, "That which doesn't kill me, makes me stronger," reminding me that I was indeed coping. The German philosopher Nietzsche sure knew what he was talking about!

Find Ways to Reduce Your Stress

A number of stress reduction techniques, such as meditation, yoga, relaxation tapes, and biofeedback, can help induce tranquility and a sense of control. You may even be able to engage in some of these while at work.

Besides their physical benefits (such as calming your breathing and releasing muscle tension), stress reduction techniques can make you more aware of changes in your body. This can help create a positive cycle: once you note the signs of stress, you can apply the technique and allow your mind to help you regain control over your body. You're back in charge. I believe the awareness of stress may be more significant than the technique you use to alleviate it.

Relaxation techniques may not provide a permanent solution to your problems, just a respite. Sometimes you may have to settle for less. Temporary stress relief may come in many forms:

- Going to a shopping mall, church, or beauty shop
- Taking a long drive into the country or to the ocean
- Smashing a tennis ball against a wall
- Listening to some quiet music
- While you're alone in the car, letting out that scream that had been building up inside you.

If you can't get out, simply taking a long bath or shower or even spending a day in bed, sleeping as your body dictates, may help. Be creative. Remember, the purpose of this activity is to get you through the moment.

My daughter wrote poetry to help her cope with her anxiety prior to her second heart surgery. After she died, I found among her things a notebook filled with page after page of incomplete poems. All revealed her deepest thoughts and fears about the danger she was facing. By the time she entered the hospital, however, she was incredibly calm. I understood why when I read the last line of the only poem she had completed:

MY HELP COMETH FROM THE LORD
The sun beats upon my back,
My body dry,
Water, water.
But none, —sand, heat, hell;

My body bends,
My lips quiver,
God, water!
My camel stops;
He kneels.
My help cometh from the Lord.
Water in the distance,
Closer, closer,
The water disappeared;
The land is dry.
My help cometh from the Lord,
My heart slows down,
Thump . . . thump . . .
Silence prevails;
My thirst is quenched.

Counseling can be a useful stress-reducer if you're so inclined. Even the strongest among us need help from time to time. Many people are uncomfortable with counseling, however, fearing it means they are out of control. If you believe counseling is not for you, be sure to recognize when you feel stressed, and do what you can to relieve it. For those who can accept it, counseling can prove eminently valuable, especially if you find a trained professional.

Ask your physician or medical social worker for a referral to a therapist who specializes in patients with chronic illnesses. Disease-oriented groups such as the American Cancer Society may also have lists of counselors who are well acquainted with the issues you are facing. In choosing a professional, be sure that you find someone with whom you can establish a warm rapport. Much emotional healing takes place within the relationship.

Should you rely on tranquilizers to reduce stress? If your doctor or you feel these medications are necessary, then perhaps you should take them. Just be aware that tranquilizers help you to relax artificially—they do not help you to come to terms with or solve your problems. They mask feelings that may otherwise need to be processed and so may interfere with your grieving your losses and eventually taking charge.

I wish I had known this when doctors tranquilized me in their effort to help me cope with the extreme stress of my daughter's death. During the nine-year period following her second surgery and death, various medications controlled my emotions. When I stopped taking them, however, I still had to undergo the grieving process. The tranquilizers delayed the resolution that might have occurred earlier.

In their heightened state of anxiety, Tom and Sally might have reached for tranquilizers. Instead, they faced their problems head-on. In so doing, Tom realized that he could not control his disease but he could control his life, while Sally learned that even strong people who are accustomed to being in control of their lives sometimes need outside help.

Evaluate Whom You Can Count On

As Tom, Sally, and I explored the many changes in diet, income, and roles that they would encounter, and they came up with alternative plans with which they felt they could live, we reached a thorny subject: To whom could they turn in the event of a medical emergency? On whom could they count among those closest to them: parents, relatives, friends, neighbors? This was particularly painful because it required that they examine all of their relationships honestly. This discussion was bound to bring up old hurts, and it did!

We began with parents. Tom had been estranged from his since his marriage to Sally—they had disapproved of her. Although Sally wanted to heal the rift, Tom was adamant: he could never count on them, so he excluded them.

Sally's parents were divorced. Sally's mother, the most available person in the family, irritated Tom. Although this couple needed help, they decided that they didn't want the assistance of someone who would add to their stress. Sally trusted and respected her dad above all the other family members, but he traveled constantly. Sally's grandmother, while well loved and nearby, was ill herself and unlikely to survive many more years.

When Tom and Sally had reviewed everyone, including their closest friends, they discovered that they could count on their neighbors the Smiths the most. In previous emergencies, this wonderful, caring couple had taken in their son, handling the situation sensitively. Tom and Sally perceived the Smiths as being good parents, an extremely important asset. By determining whom they could depend on in an emergency, Tom and Sally were preparing themselves for future shocks in an important way.

To make sure that they felt ready for all eventualities, Tom and Sally sat down with the Smiths one evening. Tom said, "Jane and Roger, we really appreciate how you've helped us in the past when we've had medical emergencies and the sensitive way you took care of Joshua. We hope that we could count on you in the event of future emergencies." The Smiths were happy to agree to this arrangement.

If you are feeling alone, you may find it beneficial to draw a chart showing upon whom you can rely for support. List everyone you feel close to or think would be there for you in case of an emergency. Then, next to each name write how you believe that person would be helpful, how available he is, the extent of his commitment to you, and how deep his resources run. You may be surprised with what you find. At the very least, this exercise can be reassuring.

Be Flexible and Creative

As a result of their careful step-by-step process, Tom and Sally were able to alleviate their own anxiety. The man who had earlier declared, "Lupus is directing my life," understood how he could wrest control away from his disease. Then, his doctor threw him another hot handle.

One day, Tom walked into my office completely crestfallen. His doctors told him that he would have to cancel his plans to go to the beach with his family that summer. Given the powerful medication he was taking, it was dangerous for him to be exposed to sunlight.

While Tom had somehow been able to cope with all of the changes he'd had to make, he called this one the last straw. The beach vacation symbolized to him the one last pleasure that had remained unchanged by his disease. Now even this was going to be taken away. Tom was devastated.

Trying to understand why this particular activity was so meaningful to Tom, I learned that he usually planned this annual event a year in advance. Their closest friends—a couple who shared their love for food, drink, and mostly talk—always accompanied them. It was a chance to recharge their collective batteries. Now Tom would lose this irreplaceable opportunity for fun and camaraderie.

Searching through my stockpile of clinical techniques to help Tom with this additional loss in his life, I realized that what he valued most about his beach vacations was being with his family and friends, preparing wonderful meals, and talking the night away. None of these activities required sun. I asked, "Would you be willing to go to the beach and stay in the house all day?"

At first, Tom was puzzled by this strange, almost contradictory question. After a few minutes, as he began to realize what I was asking, a smile brightened his face. "Yes," he said emphatically, "of course, I can stay out of the sun." He was ecstatic because this new arrangement would preserve what he loved best about his vacations.

"Look," I said, "before you make any final decisions, ask your doctors whether this is safe for you." I felt sure they would grant his request. After all, if he didn't go and he remained depressed, they would have to consider what effect this would have on his physical condition. And they did.

Sally called the next day to report the good news. They had won the psychological battle over Tom's disease. "Lupus has deprived him of so many important things in his life," Sally said, "but it hasn't deprived him of everything!"

A year after this couple had completed their treatment with me, I received a letter from them. As I opened the envelope, a photo fell out onto my desk. It was a picture of a new, modern beach house they had just built with an inheritance. It was clearly a symbol of Tom's victory in his struggle with his disease.

Sally and Tom had to grapple with life-and-death decisions when they first came to me. But as a result of the basic life changes they made, they were subsequently able to roll with the punches. Tom was grateful to be alive. He was willing to try anything to hang on to whatever small part of his former life-style he could salvage. Such an attitude takes a commitment to live and enjoy what you can. Once you pledge to yourself to be open, flexible, and creative, you can find solutions to problems that might have once seemed insoluble.

Join Support Groups

Sometimes it helps to know that you are not alone with your problems. You may feel comforted by realizing that others struggle with similar issues and that there are places for you to find support. Your community may have a local chapter of national health organizations, such as the American Cancer Society, the American Heart Association, the Lupus Foundation of America, the Cystic Fibrosis Foundation, or the National Multiple Sclerosis Society. Your telephone directory, local hospital, or toll-free phone information number (800-555-1212) can help you locate an organization that represents your ailment.

These associations offer the latest medical information and often have peer support groups. The latter are composed of people like you; who share your disease and the practical and emotional consequences resulting from it. These participants can be objective with you because they are strangers, but empathic because they have encountered the problems firsthand, in a way that your family and friends have not.

Knowing that others experience the same frightening feelings as you do and are possibly struggling even harder than you to control them, can put your problems into a broader perspective. Family groups are also often available, since families frequently need more support than ill people (see chapter 3).

Plan Ahead

When you minimize surprises, you stay in better control of situations. This is true in a mundane way as well as globally. Therefore, I believe it wise to do a little planning and scouting. What an unwelcome surprise to leave the restaurant dinner table, for example, only to discover that you cannot maneuver the steep flight of stairs to get to the rest rooms! Knowing in advance the location of the rest rooms will help you avoid panic later. Call in advance to learn about handicap accessibility.

If you cannot get to the bathroom on time and do have an accident, you can rehearse what you will say to others around you. You might make a joke of the situation, saying, "It's uncomfortable squishing around in wet shoes," or straight forwardly as in, "I have MS and can't always make it to the bathroom on time." Or, you can simply express your embarrassment. Even simple plans such as these can help you remain in charge of your life.

Plan for future activities you may enjoy: vacations, books to read, classes. On a broader scope and if you feel comfortable doing so, you and your family may wish to plan for the future. For example, you might want to arrange for the care of your children or elderly parents should you become incapacitated. Or after a serious discussion, your spouse may decide to return to school, in preparation for becoming the chief breadwinner in the family.

Of course, some people feel uncomfortable planning so far in advance, especially when it comes to major life issues. Nevertheless, others do need the sense of control in order to feel safe. Recognize what your needs are. If you feel better making plans, then by all means do it!

Use the Power of the Mind

Never underestimate the power of this simple expression: "feeling better." In *Anatomy of an Illness as Perceived by the Patient*, former *Saturday Review* editor Norman Cousins explained how laughter and pleasant thoughts shooed away his blues and affected his physical state. Cousins and a host of other researchers and authors have discovered that the mind is a powerful weapon just waiting to be used to your benefit. It can decrease stress and even heal the body.

It is particularly sad, therefore, to encounter patients who remain stuck in their negative fantasies, picturing the worst that can happen to them and acting accordingly. They adhere to these gloomy thoughts, no matter what, repeating them like a broken record. If you find yourself in this painful situation, you must first recognize that you are in the doldrums and then discover some way to pull yourself out. You might want to read a book, call a friend, watch a comedy on TV, take a walk, pull some weeds—whatever you can to cheer yourself up.

Although this tendency has diminished with the passage of years, I still sometimes wonder what my life would have been like if two of my children hadn't become ill and died. (Certainly, I wouldn't have written this book!) I spin around on this old track for a while and then give myself a good hard mental shake. "Irene," I say to myself, "this isn't useful. That's not what happened. You can't replay your life. Don't waste any more precious time and energy on wishes that cannot come true. It's better to use your life to make the most of what you do have."

Certainly, it's not bad or wrong to wish or fantasize. Sometimes the activity is useful; it helps to bring life into perspective. You don't have to fear your negative thoughts, only manage them and keep them in control. The key here is to recognize what you're doing and why, and then give yourself a nudge and move on.

No one has all the answers, and no one can anticipate all the problems he or she will face in life, long-term illness or not. Still, the mind has power over the body—although it can activate anxiety, it may also generate hopeful and joyous thoughts, creating positive energy that helps you restore a sense of control. Once your initial anxiety lifts, you'll be surprised at how well you know how to manage. Trust yourself!

REMEMBER

- Your long-term illness may make you feel as if you've lost control over your life.
- You may feel disoriented.
- Although you may not be able to control your body, you can control your mind and how you respond to your disease.

THINGS TO DO

- Separate the immediate problems from the long-term ones.
- Make your own decisions wherever possible.
- Evaluate and change what's changeable.
- Pinpoint areas of stress.
- Set reachable and reasonable goals that help reduce stress.
- Salvage what you can of old coping mechanisms.
- Use stress reduction techniques.
- Evaluate to whom you can turn when the going gets rough.
- Be flexible and creative.
- Join support groups.
- Plan ahead.
- Use the power of your mind.

6.

Mastering Your Fear of Loss of Self-Image

Your self-image or sense of self is composed of many physical and personality traits. These include your:

- Appearance and attractiveness
- Alertness and intellectual abilities
- Stamina and strength
- Family relationships
- Role as husband or wife, son or daughter, father or mother
- Health and vitality
- Friendliness
- Productivity and career trajectory
- Financial position
- Capacity to give of yourself and express affection
- Sexuality and ability to bear children
- View of the world
- Spirituality and belief in God.

Your long-term illness may affect any and all of these: once diagnosed, you may no longer view yourself as the same person. What was once familiar is now lost. Indeed, a change of identity is a common and natural, albeit painful, outgrowth of your condition. Yet surprisingly, it can also be a source of great personal growth. In this chapter, I'll show you how.

THE CONSEQUENCES OF LOSS OF SELF-IMAGE

Your disease has already delivered a powerful physical blow—now it lands an emotional one as well. The loss of self-image strikes deep into the heart of who you are, who you have always been, and who you might become.

You may feel as if you're floating in a state of suspended identity formation. Having recently lost your old sense of self, you may not yet have formed a new one with which to replace it. You may be aware that you now face uncharted waters, but are mystified as to how you will navigate them. Shortly after diagnosis, almost everyone experiences this dilemma and the intense anxiety that it provokes.

Unfortunately, this can have a detrimental effect on your state of mind and your relationship with others. When your anxiety level increases, all the fears you may have developed during your lifetime (that you're "unlovable," that you're "clumsy," that you're "worthless") surface in an exaggerated manner. I call these "ghosts." When you are highly stressed, as you most likely are after diagnosis, you can almost count on their appearing to haunt you!

Because of these ghosts, the change in self-image affects not only how you feel about yourself, but also how others may respond to you. That's because people *project* their self-image. When you feel good about yourself, you unconsciously send out positive signals: there's a smile on your lips, a lilt in your voice, and a spring in your step. Your eyes shine with excitement and you exude confidence.

People whom you encounter read such body language and react positively. Strangers will approach you in a crowded room, just to talk. Fellow pedestrians will smile and nod as you pass on the street. Perhaps shoppers in a supermarket will approach you, asking embarrassedly, "Do you know where they keep the canned corn in this place?"

On the other hand, when you're anxious and your ghosts prevail, you emit more negative signals: your eyes appear dull and downcast, your brow furrowed, your hands and jaw clenched, your neck and shoulders tight. You seem absorbed in your own thoughts, detached, in another world. Under these circumstances, you may find that a saleswoman responds to your questions gruffly, or the policeman who has stopped you gives you a ticket.

Even worse, when you're feeling miserable and need positive feedback, people may turn away and stay away. That's the last thing you want. Indeed, it becomes a vicious circle. The unhappier you feel, the more you project your gloom, and the further away others stay. This, of course, increases your misery index, and on it goes.

AM I A "SICK" PERSON?

How you resolve your identity crisis may depend on the progress of your disease and the manifestation of its symptoms—for instance, the repercussions of a stroke can be immediate and obvious, whereas the consequences of diabetes may take years to materialize.

If your illness strikes suddenly and virulently, you may have to recognize that your life is now changed forever. On the other hand, if you have a condition that develops slowly, you may find yourself in a state of limbo, unsure of whether you are "sick" or "well." In fact, although you may have been told that you have a serious disorder, in the early stages it may not take the dramatic form you expected. Perhaps you missed only a few days of work and feel relatively well. You may begin thinking, "This isn't as bad as I thought. I'm not so sick. I can handle this."

Then one morning, you may awaken and find that your hand is trembling or that your mouth has become distorted. You feel shocked. Alarmed, you call your physician. He predicts that the problem will disappear within a few hours. He's correct. In a short while your body does return to its normal state. But during those few hours, you are once again brought face-to-face with the harsh realities of your illness. You no longer wonder whether you're sick: the truth is inescapable. Lo and behold, the very next day, you're back at work as if nothing had happened.

Inhabiting this limbo between sickness and health is emotionally and physically taxing. Your hopes are high one day and dashed the next. When you're feeling well, you make plans, your emotional energy soars, you feel physically strong and able to perform normal activities. But when your symptoms reappear, your energy becomes blocked. You feel exhausted, dizzy, unable to think clearly. You must change your plans against your will. You can hardly remember how well you felt the day before; and you wonder how you were crazy enough to undertake such an ambitious project in the first place. Yesterday, you felt the whole world was before you; today you feel beaten down.

However, in the course of taking charge, you will come to accept that your view of yourself will now be different. As you relinquish your old identity and embrace an altered one, you eventually understand that *you may be "sick," but you are also functional.*

In working with the chronically ill, I have found that there are three stages to adopting this new, more realistic self-image. You must:

1. Grieve your losses.
2. Let go of your old identity.
3. Forge a new self-image.

These steps take time. Don't let anyone push you to adapt faster than you are comfortable. There's no timetable here. Each person goes through this process at her own pace. Now let's look at these steps in more detail.

Grieving Your Losses

You must give yourself permission to grieve your losses: to cry, to lament, to mourn. Often, we think we can bypass this painful process so basic to healing. Ascribing to the theory that "time heals all wounds," we believe that if we plunge ourselves into work or projects, our problems will take care of themselves.

Time can heal a physical injury. We feel a scab tingle, pull, and draw as it mends. We know that in a week or a month it will be gone, save for a scar. But mental wounds are not so simple. They may hurt throughout the body and mind. In order to grieve your losses, you must allow yourself to feel the pain and know that it will pass. Rather than running from this process by occupying yourself with activities, you must reach into your pain and give yourself over to it. Treat this as an opportunity to retreat and retrench. If you don't, your losses and change of self-image can remain unresolved for many years and can return to haunt you as new ghosts.

Moreover, although a change in identity may seem remote because symptoms may have not yet manifested themselves, if you've been told you have a long-term illness, chances are you will feel differently about yourself. In fact, one day you may look in the mirror and think, "Gee, I still look like my old self but I know that I'm changed. There's a part of me that's gone. I'm not the same person I

was. I don't know yet if it's good or bad, but I'm different!"
Your self-confidence will be threatened.

The strongest and most succinct statement of this
altered self-perception sprang from the lips of my client
Rebecca, a thirty-five-year-old woman with endometriosis.
A few weeks after her diagnosis, this bright, articulate jour-
nalist walked into my office and declared, "I'm damaged
goods!"

I have found that Rebecca's is a near universal experience. Almost all the people who have sought my help have
expressed similar painful thoughts. Their feeling of being
irreversibly flawed colors every aspect of their lives: their
work, friendships, family relationships, and sexuality.
Here are some of the statements they have made to me
over the years:

- "I feel ugly and unattractive."
- "My body is disfigured. Who will ever find me sexy?"
- "I have become awkward and clumsy."
- "I am less capable, less interesting, less valued than I used to be."
- "I'm afraid I'm no longer interesting to my friends."
- "I'm afraid my spouse will seek other partners."

You, like so many other people with chronic illness, may
experience these profoundly unsettling thoughts. You may
become caught in a struggle between longing for a return to
the person you once were and a fear of whom you might
become. In fact, you are grieving your losses.

THE LOSSES YOU MAY FACE

Everyone over the age of five or six diagnosed with a long-
term illness will experience this process of loss and reiden-
tification. Sometimes it requires a major effort, especially if
one puts great store in physical strength or appearance. The

furniture mover who can no longer lift the refrigerator, the model who must abandon leg-flattering high heels, and the dancer who needs a cane to walk all face profound challenges as they alter the way they think of themselves. Consider how you feel about physical impairment.

The same, of course, is also true of diminished mental capacity, but you can be prepared. Grant was diagnosed with Alzheimer's disease in the early stages. A naval engineer, he had been trained to be precise in his thinking. He came to me to grieve his future losses. Then, knowing what lay in store for him, he adapted in his realistic way. He considered all the tasks that might be difficult for him in the future and arranged for others to handle them. He had long discussions with his daughter about what she should do in the event of his mental impairment.

You may also grieve the loss of your productivity. Many individuals value themselves in relation to their work. When illness forces them into a premature retirement, they feel worthless—bereft of their purpose in life and usefulness to their families. Productivity can also mean the capacity to sire or bear children. Impotence and/or sterility are a great blow to a man, as is a woman's inability to conceive and carry a pregnancy to term. Indeed, one of my patients lamented that losing her reproductive organs and no longer having the possibility of bearing children were more upsetting to her than her cancer diagnosis.

But be careful not to confuse grieving with blaming. Don't blame your illness on weaknesses in your personality. You're dealing with quite enough already! To believe that somehow you have caused your illness is counterproductive and can be destructive, especially when you are trying everything possible to live with your disease. All your energy should now go toward taking charge, not blaming yourself.

In truth, your personality—essentially you—did not cause the ailment: nature, your genes, and/or your environment did. Besides, no one wants a chronic condition. Lisa, for example, believed that she had triggered her breast cancer because her work as a policewoman made her highly stressed and intense. Her assumption was untrue. I pointed out to her that her colleagues, working under similar difficult conditions, did not become ill. In this way I persuaded her that she should let go of the additional burden of being angry with herself. It was depriving her of vital energy she needed to fight her disease.

List your losses as a result of your disease. Here's what Jerold, a patient of mine suffering from cardiovascular problems and high blood pressure, came up with:

1. Difficulty with erection due to medication
2. No more steak and eggs for breakfast
3. No more smoking
4. Can't jog anymore
5. Have to buy special, unsalted foods and no bacon
6. Can't just order off the menu at restaurants.

Save your list of losses both great and small. We'll be working with it later.

Letting Go

After you have given yourself permission to grieve your losses, you can move on to the next phase: letting go of your old self-image. This is no easy task. Your pre-illness identity is the only one you've ever had and giving it up can cause a great deal of anxiety. This is, in part, because you have not willingly sought out this change. Your illness imposed it on you. You're probably also terribly unsure of what your new self-image will be. When externally imposed change is coupled with unknowable consequences, distress can grow and grow.

If you don't know what lies ahead, if you let yourself imagine what you may become, you may conjure some extremely frightening images. To counteract your fears, you might find it helpful to allow these terrifying thoughts to come to the surface—for instance, by writing them down on a piece of paper. This is a way to rid yourself of these thoughts by getting them off your mind. After you've had a chance to clear your head, you may want to crumple up the paper and throw it away.

While you are writing down your fears, you will notice that your thoughts are just that—thoughts. Facing down your worst fears, privately or with someone you trust, will help you release the tension they create. You needn't be ashamed of them. They are all legitimate and normal. It may seem contradictory to describe terror as commonplace, but consider whether you could respond in any other way, given that you're facing an uncertain future.

As you go through this process, you may feel the need for support, particularly from a sympathetic ear. A peer support group can be quite helpful at this time (see pp. 108–109 on how to locate one). In this group, you will hear others struggling with the same issues that plague you, and you will realize that you are not alone.

Recognizing that your reaction is absolutely normal should help to reduce some of the anxiety it has created. Moreover, knowing that you are not "going crazy" or that you are not the only one to feel as you do should help to move you out of a cycle of ambivalence to a position of strength—one from which you can deal with your problems. You will no longer vacillate, but will be able to identify, understand, and master your emotions.

On the other hand, brooding about issues that you are powerless to change can sap energy you'll need to stay healthy and strong. To help you let go of these issues, make a pair of lists showing what is useless to you now and what is useful. This will clear your head of "excess baggage" by delineating those parts of your old self-image you might wish to hang on to but that in fact no longer serve any useful purpose. This exercise will help you prioritize your thinking. You will recognize what is valuable to you in your new life and let go of what is no longer relevant.

For example, my patient Alice had gained quite a few pounds as a result of chemotherapy after breast cancer surgery. It was *useless* for her to lament her lost girlish figure, since she needed the medication to increase her chances of survival. It was *useful,* on the other hand, for this woman to activate her sense of style. Alice maintained her attractive appearance by shopping for some new clothes. She purchased several outfits and accessories that flattered her new, temporarily larger body. What follows is a sample of Alice's useless/useful list:

USELESS	USEFUL
1. Worry about weight	1. Wear clothes that minimize size
2. Upset about no menstruation	2. Enjoy sex more freely
3. Scar shows with low décolletage	3. Wear higher necklines, scarves, and jewelry
4. Dismay about swollen arm.	4. Wear attractive, long-sleeved blouses.

This list helped Alice to focus on her strengths rather than the deficits her illness had created.

Forging a New Self-Image

Does the prospect of creating a "new you" sound like a tall order? Wait! Maybe the changes are neither as all encompassing nor as difficult to cope with as you anticipate. Parts of your old identity not only may remain intact but may become your greatest assets. As a result of your condition you may sustain major physical losses but may grow in new ways.

Look at what happened to Sam. When he fell ill with leukemia, he knew that he would no longer be able to play basketball with his friends. As he became more home-bound, he discovered that his pals still enjoyed his company. In fact, he began seeing his buddies more often than before, and his home became a fun meeting place.

If you are willing to go through the process of self-examination, you may discover that the vacuum caused by any losses will allow other, previously unexplored traits to come to the fore. For example, although Sam had always disdained quiet activities, he discovered that he could actually enjoy conversations about politics and sports. He even had more time to read. Moreover, previously, he had done very little entertaining at home, but now he looked forward to the camaraderie and to planning meals for his buddies. He found that people not only enjoyed his hospitality, but also his delightful, newly emergent personality traits.

Take pride in your real strengths. In an exercise earlier in this chapter, I asked you to list what you have lost as a result of your illness. Now, list what you still possess—traits that can never be taken away: your warm smile; your sense of caring about others; your perseverance; your intelligence and curiosity; your ability to organize, think logically, and reason, to make judgments, to be a good friend and listener.

Examine your weaknesses as well as your strengths. You might be surprised to learn that often these traits are relative. For example, if you make spur-of-the-moment decisions it may mean that you are impulsive and haven't thought situations through carefully, or it may mean that you are unafraid to take action when you must. Keeping your illness in mind, you might chart your weaknesses in one column and your strengths in another. Imagine them in play in different situations at home or at work.

What you consider a weakness in one environment (bossiness at home) may be a strength in another (assertiveness at work). You may ask yourself the following questions: Is it good now for me to be less bossy at home and more assertive at work? Since my family is spending more time doing things for me, is it more appropriate for me to be less demanding? You may not be changing your self, but you may wish to change some of your behavior.

Next, "try on" various new "selves" until you find one that fits. You might make another chart to help you explore untried options. Again, referring to your list of losses (see p. 120), write a possible substitution next to each item. For example, if you can't jog anymore you may be able to substitute swimming or walking. These alternatives may seem a poor replacement for the original, but in time, you may realize their value. You may, for example, have to give up the hecticness of a globe-trotting career, as did Tom, the man with lupus in chapter 5, but you may be rewarded with a satisfying, slower-paced life-style that provides you with many more productive years. As you go through this exercise, you will realize that *your new identity will be based on strengths you currently possess rather than on those you now lack.*

Once you have confronted your feelings, you will project yourself more positively. Your behavior acts as a beacon to those around you, signaling to them how you would like to be treated. Even if you're confined to a wheelchair, you can make aggressive eye contact, ask questions, and project your voice. One of my young patients in a wheelchair became a cheerleader at her school. "I like myself, so you can like me too," was her clear message.

HELPING YOUR FAMILY ADJUST

All her life, Francine had known her father to be a strong, positive, and successful surgeon; Harold had run the surgical team at a large hospital with authority and aplomb. After a moderately debilitating stroke, he became in Francine's words, "passive, weak, and submissive." He depended entirely on his wife for care and even for simple day-to-day decision making.

"I can't get over the change in him," Francine confided during a counseling session. "I've been shocked and disappointed. I've pressed him to be more active. I'll say, 'Dad, wouldn't it be easier if you shaved yourself today?' but he just rebuffs my attempts to engage him in even the most basic elements of grooming himself."

Unfortunately, Francine didn't understand that her father had not yet adapted to his altered condition. Harold could no longer present his old self-image, but he had not created a new one to replace what was lost. How much easier it might have been for both of them had he articulated his feelings to his loving but frustrated daughter. He could have told her what role he wanted to play now and what identity he wished to assume. That would have eased Francine's anxiety considerably. But as it stood, neither father nor daughter had processed the changes caused by the stroke.

As you undergo your own self-evaluation and transformation, consider that your family must also undergo a similar experience. Just as you make adjustments, so must your loved ones. They too may feel anxiety about your new personality traits. Their self-images may change as well while they integrate shifts in your identity. Everyone's feelings need to be aired in order for the transformation to proceed (see chapter 3).

If you have taken charge of your life, you can help your loved ones through the adjustment process. You might find the following suggestions helpful:

1. Explain to your family that you are reconciling yourself to a new self-image. You feel different about who you are and need time to integrate what has happened to you.

2. Reassure them that you understand their need to find a new equilibrium too. You are all going through a rough time together.

3. Give your family the time and space to pinpoint and grieve their own losses. You might suggest that they read this chapter and do the exercises, to help them understand what you're going through and deal with their own shifting identities.

4. Recognize that what feels good for your spouse or family may be uncomfortable for you now and vice versa. You need to give your loved ones the opportunity to adjust to the new reality. Inform them of your feelings. If you believe they are pressing you to go out with friends too soon, or to call coworkers when you're still feeling upset and tentative, you can say "I still feel shaky this week. Maybe next week. I do appreciate your pushing me. I know you care, but I'm not quite ready."

MAKING A NEW LIFE

I'd like to share with you the progress my patient Louise made as she came to grips with her diagnosis of multiple sclerosis. Louise's story demonstrates that it is possible to create a rewarding life even when parts of your identity have changed as a result of a long-term illness.

Louise, a young law school graduate, was another of my patients who saw herself as "damaged goods." For several months after her diagnosis, she had been preoccupied with physical needs: CAT scans, medication, bed rest. The tests indicated that her case was relatively mild. Now that she required less medical attention, she was able to focus on her mental status, and frankly, it wasn't all that good. In fact, when she appeared in my office, this young woman described herself as being at the lowest point in her life.

A pressing problem had brought Louise's mental health into focus: her bar exam was only several weeks away. She had to find a way to muster the physical stamina required for four days of testing and the mental agility to answer legendarily difficult questions. "I'm depressed and anxious," she confided during our first session. "I'm not my old confident self anymore. I just don't know how I'm going to get through those exams."

Louise feared for herself if she didn't pass the bar. It represented to her the culmination of four years of grueling work: she had attended law school at night while holding down a full-time job. "If I fail because of this sickness, after waiting and working so long and so hard, I'll just die," she sobbed. "Everything I've worked for and hoped to achieve will be lost. I'm terrified of the future."

Listening to Louise's tale of woe, I felt sure that I could help her through this dreaded exam. But based on her "damaged goods" self-assessment, I wasn't so sure how she would fare the rest of her life.

From the busy schedule she had kept before her illness, it was clear to me that Louise was a hardworking individual who enjoyed overcoming challenges. She relished doing several things at once and always worked with a high level of energy. Now, however, in order for her to get through the bar exam, Louise was going to have to learn to pace herself. That would help her conserve her physical energy so that she could direct it to the task at hand—the exam. Pacing also meant that she would probably need to take ten-minute rest breaks every hour, which would require a special dispensation from the examiners.

But before Louise could apply for this kind of assistance, she had to overcome a psychological hurdle. The idea of pacing herself didn't sit well with her. "Only elderly and handicapped people need to do that," she complained. Indeed, if she accepted the fact that she had to slow down, she would also have to recognize that she had become a different person—she was "sick."

Still, Louise's desire to pass the bar was stronger than her reluctance to integrate this new identity. As she listened to my explanation, she saw the practicality of it. Pacing oneself is a good technique for anyone—healthy or ill. I not only offered her the possibility of making the most of her limited energy, but also held out the hope of generating more energy. With few other options available, Louise accepted this premise and eagerly learned some relaxation techniques and other commonsense ideas, including getting enough sleep and eating more healthfully.

Louise was an excellent student—both of the law and of self-pacing. She reported on how my suggestions had helped her through the exams. Later she learned that she had passed the bar with flying colors. Based on this success, Louise announced her desire to work on a difficult personal problem: her relationships with men. These had always been problematic for her, and now that she was ill, she was sure she would never find someone to love.

"I've always felt unfeminine, unattractive, and clumsy," she explained. "But now, with the prospect of shaky hands, wheelchairs, and canes, who would want me? I'll never get married and have children." These issues made the bar exam pale in comparison.

As we explored the problems more deeply, I came to see that one of Louise's ghosts was her fear of being unappealing to men. She had dated, but as soon as a man became interested in her, she turned him off with her overeagerness to please. Rather than allowing the man to court her, she raced past this important stage in the relationship and immediately tried to establish intimacy. She made the follow-up calls, bought the special event tickets, or invited him to home-cooked gourmet meals. As a result, the man soon lost interest, often failing to return her increasingly anxious calls.

Louise's story was particularly heartbreaking because she was attractive, bright, fun, and multitalented. She was successful in all her other relationships, enjoying a large and varied group of friends in whose company she was relaxed and confident, and adored by her family.

Searching for the reason that Louise was so successful with some people and so unsuccessful with others, I discovered that as a child, in an attempt to compensate for feeling unattractive, Louise had always tried to be "good." She believed that only if she were "good" enough—perpetually giving, helpful, caring—would others love her. As a result, Louise became a caretaker. Most of the people in her life rewarded her for this behavior, but it didn't serve her well with men who needed to be in charge during the early stages of the relationship.

Louise also had to consider her need to be a caretaker in light of her illness. What if, one day, she had to be the receiver of care rather than the giver? It was vital for Louise to understand her ghost.

Now came the hard part of the work. Louise had to look back on the foundation of her old perceptions, relationships, and values. She needed to ask herself difficult questions. Where did she get her ideas about being "unattractive"? Did she have to be "sexy" in order for a man to love her? What about her feeling of being "damaged goods"—did these thoughts come from people close to her or from her own mind? Were "shaky hands, wheelchairs, and canes" more frightening to them or to her?

Once Louise understood the source of her perceptions, she could test how others felt about her. She had to be sure how she felt about being physically disabled and clear on how much any future marriage would actually depend on her physical abilities. If the negative perceptions were hers, then she could change them. If they came from those around her, she would have to tell or show them more about herself, so that they too could alter their attitudes.

It was difficult for Louise to confront the frightening possibility of future disability, especially since her symptoms were still minimal. But in examining her thoughts she discovered that no one else in her world considered her "funny looking" except for her!

One point I had hoped would become clear for Louise (which eventually did) was the distinction between "love" and "sexiness." "Sexy" is a relative term. Some men like fragile women while others like those with high energy. Indeed, I have found that some husbands and boyfriends of my female MS patients found their mates increasingly sexually appealing, even as they became less stable. What was embarrassing for these women was exhilarating for their men! Perhaps their increased dependence or vulnerability was arousing.

As Louise readied herself to put her new self-awareness into action, she faced a few more challenges. She had to grieve the losses she had incurred as a result of her disease and also value the abilities that remained. Yes, she had lost some physical strength. She told me she might never play tennis again, but she had never played much anyway. As we continued this line of thought, she realized that tennis didn't matter all that much to most men anyway. She still had more than enough strength to work, socialize, make love, and have babies.

We also concluded that although there was some damage to her body, her mind was still intact. She could always practice law and maintain her friendships. At the end of this arduous process, Louise learned that it was her old self-image that had made her feel unlovable, not the multiple sclerosis. Her new identity would be based on what she had—not what she lacked.

Once Louise was able to grow into this more positive view of herself, wonderful changes came into her life. She met a "perfect" man who fell head over heels in love with her. They married; a few years later, I received the first of several birth announcements.

In her letters to me over the years, it has become clear that no matter how physically limited she might become, Louise will always be a giving person. It was this quality that had endeared her to all who knew her, including her husband. She has become helpful to him in practical ways too. He has political aspirations, and she has many fine political skills. Perhaps most important, she can always provide him with unfailing personal support. Her best quality—her ability to be a good friend—will never be destroyed by her disease.

The changes in Louise's life occurred because she underwent a difficult and painful self-evaluation and learned to adopt a new identity based on her strengths. She took a plunge into deep, uncharted waters, but swam gracefully to the surface. She had my assistance, but her fortitude brought her through. It wasn't that she was such a willing diver—it's just that the alternatives were so much less appealing!

REMEMBER

- You are in the process of changing your identity. This is normal.
- You may feel a great deal of anxiety at this time. Your anxiety may awaken old fears—your ghosts.
- You project good and bad feelings about yourself.
- Your family and friends need time to adjust to the new you. They may even need to alter their own identities.
- A change of identity can be painful but it can also promote personal growth.

THINGS TO DO

- Examine how you perceived yourself in the past and now. How do you feel about physical impairment?
- List and grieve your losses.
- Measure your strengths and weaknesses.
- Let go of attributes or issues that are no longer useful to you.
- Forge a new identity based on your strengths.
- Ask your family and friends to be partners in your efforts to change behavior.
- Get professional support if you need it or join a peer support group. You don't have to go it alone.

7.

Mastering Your Fear of Dependency

Marion required professional help to become an independent woman once more. A psychiatrist referred her to me after he had tried but failed to lift her out of a three-year depression following a debilitating stroke.

Physically, seventy-year-old Marion had recovered almost completely. She had rehabilitated her stricken right arm and leg, and although she spoke haltingly and her voice had a strange timbre, she had regained most of her ability to communicate. She was able to think as clearly as before, but her mouth and tongue muscles wouldn't respond as quickly as she wanted them to. Her biggest problems were now psychological.

Several months after her stroke, Marion and her husband, Larry, had moved into a new, smaller home in a retirement community. Now, some two and a half years later, she had still to unpack the moving boxes. She refused to participate in other activities that were central to her life before her illness: for instance, she no longer left her house, she would not cook, and she shunned old, dear friends.

Meeting Marion for the first time, I realized she had no idea why she had remained depressed for such a long time. She had regained most of her former faculties and strength, and she had great personal support: Larry had given up his public relations business to care for her. But she still couldn't get her life back together again.

While I initially met with Marion and Larry as a couple, I soon realized that whenever I asked Marion a question, her husband would answer it. I could see that he was trying to protect her and was compensating for her speech difficulties. However, by speaking for her, Larry had unwittingly postponed Marion's recovery. His well-intentioned act was preventing her from regaining her old self-confidence in speaking. She would have to do that before she could emerge from her depression.

I noted that even as Larry pushed and prodded Marion to be her former, lively self, he prevented her from struggling with her problems and overcoming them on her own. The more he hovered, the more dependent and insecure she became. Each time he encouraged her to do something she had once enjoyed, he unwittingly intensified her feelings that she would never live up to his expectations—she would never be the woman she had been—and she withdrew even more. Of course, this was the opposite of the independent woman he so desperately wanted her to be again.

I soon arranged to see Marion and Larry separately. During our time alone, Marion described her formerly strong independent spirit. This was a trait that she and her husband had valued. "I loved chopping wood and carrying it back to the house without Larry's help," she boasted.

For his part, Larry had come to depend on Marion's self-reliance. "My work required that I travel, sometimes for months at a time. Even though we lived in an isolated house, tucked deep in the woods, I never worried about Marion. I was always confident that she could take care of herself, and she always did."

Marion's autonomy was based on her exceptionally strong mind and body. Prior to her stroke, at age sixty-seven, she had had great physical robustness. Her stubborn independence of mind, a quality she had used well in her many community involvements had been equally robust. She had created and run several organizations. In addition, she had had a gift for words; she loved public speaking and did it often.

In fact, it was Marion's verbal abilities that Larry mourned most. With tears in his eyes, he said, "I really miss the repartee we used to share. Every night on my way home from work, I would look forward to our discussions about politics and books. Now I don't even attempt that because it's too painful to watch her struggle."

As a result of her stroke, Marion had lost—or so she believed—her greatest assets: her physical strength, her ability to communicate, and her fierce independence. It was my job to help her realize that she may have been deprived of some parts of these but that other parts—especially her cherished independence—were still within her grasp. I'll return to her story later in the chapter.

YOUR NEWLY DEPENDENT STATE

As the poet John Donne wrote hundreds of years ago, "No man is an island entire of itself." All people, whether healthy or ill, must interrelate with others, and thus struggle with the issues of independence and dependence: *What can I do for myself? How much can I or must I rely on others?*

Since long-term illnesses amplify this internal conflict, dependency issues often surface soon after diagnosis. Suddenly, you may feel totally alone; you may desperately want someone to take care of you physically and emotionally. Conversely, you may hate the idea that you are no longer autonomous, that you must depend on others now.

Whether your illness requires round-the-clock or minimal care, you will at some point come face-to-face with your dependency needs. Indeed, at one time or another you may find that you must ask others to assist you:

- Physically: walking, turning over in bed, eating, going to the bathroom
- Financially: paying hospital and home-nursing bills, taking over as chief breadwinner, writing checks, keeping the family books
- Medically: administering medication, changing dressings, attending to proper diet
- Practically: shopping, grooming, cleaning the house, baby-sitting
- Emotionally: reassuring you and giving support when you're feeling down, holding your hand when you're in pain.

As long as you require some form of medical supervision, you will always be a "patient" and thus dependent (at least on medical personnel). Ideally, as you take charge of your life, you will become comfortable asking for help from people other than health professionals (who provide it as a matter of course), and you will learn to accept help while remaining as independent as you are able or wish to be. The goal of this chapter is to help you recognize and anticipate your fears so you can do just that.

When Dependency Is Natural and Helpful

As you leave your doctor's office immediately after diagnosis, dependency issues may be rather abstract for you. But if you must go to the hospital for treatment, your physical and emotional dependence becomes instantly concrete. There are no two ways about it: as a hospital inpatient you rely on others to take care of you. You ask the nurses for help getting up and down. They feed, bathe, and dress you, if necessary. You count on and heed the doctor's orders and wait for your food to be delivered.

Your dependence is not only appropriate, it is also vital to the success of your treatment. The more compliant, cooperative, and relaxed you are, the better your chances of healing.

Home Is a Bit More Complicated

When you go home, your role as a patient becomes less clear. To begin with, expectations change and can conflict.

- Your physician expects that now you and your family will be responsible for your care.
- Your family expects that you are better now and should be able to resume some of your former responsibilities.
- You expect that your family will care for you until you're mentally and physically ready to go out in the world again.

In the hospital, you may have had little trouble asking for help if you needed it; you might have even demanded it as your right. Yet, due to the high cost of hospital care and new insurance-company directives, these days people are leaving the hospital earlier, sicker, and thus more vulnerable than ever before. You may need more assistance at home, but asking for and receiving it may only make you feel guilty. Your spouse may be tired, for example, working two jobs to cover your medical expenses, and you may feel hard pressed to ask him to do more for you (see chapter 3).

In these circumstances, it would be wise for you and your loved ones to examine how you feel about dependency early on, as a way to forestall future conflicts (see p. 48). Going to extremes by shying away from your dependency or becoming completely dependent can be overwhelming for all of you and can invite disaster.

Besides, other tensions exist at home. Whereas in the hospital, everyone was focused on your needs, at home you may be competing with the needs of others. During a session in my office, Brad described how upset he felt about having to share his wife's attention. Late one afternoon while Lara was changing his bandages, she had to drop everything and run into the kitchen to see whether the chicken soup was boiling over.

"I realized while she was gone," he explained, "that it was only an hour to dinner and the children were already asking when it would be ready. Lara was in the kitchen for what seemed to me like an eternity. The kids must have asked her to help them with their homework. But while she left me alone, I started to worry that she hadn't cleaned the wound well. She was in such a hurry to get into the kitchen.

"She must have seen the expression on my face when she came back in the room because she asked me, 'Are you all right?' I didn't want to complain because I was afraid I would hurt her feelings. I need her help so much, it scares me."

In the hospital, the atmosphere is calm and quiet, but at home you must deal with the normal noises and confusion of a busy household. On another occasion, Brad heard his children bickering in the next room and his wife yelling at them to quiet down so he could get his rest. He thought, "Will my kids be angry at me because they're no longer free to play in their own home?" The truth was, Brad needed his children to help him around the home. He was dependent on them too and didn't want to offend them.

DEPENDENCY IS NOT A PROBLEM FOR EVERYONE

For some individuals, dependency is a natural, satisfying state. Many thrive on the extra attention they receive and even know how to make their caregiver feel valued. When interviewed on a morning radio talk show, for example, one young woman explained that caring for her seriously ill and severely disabled mother-in-law provided her with such deep satisfaction that she actually felt dependent on her mother-in-law! "I need her more than she needs me," was the way this young woman summed up their well-balanced relationship. This is the best one can hope for in the face of what can often be an exhausting and trying experience.

Melissa, a young woman in a wheelchair, rewarded her husband generously for his devotion to her by presenting him with a new poem every evening when he came home from work. She had found a way to lift his tired body and spirits at the end of each day and to let him know how much she appreciated his taking a second job to cover the extra medical expenses incurred by her illness. As dependent as Melissa was on her husband for medical and physical care, she independently provided him with a gift that only she could give.

Even if being dependent has been uncomfortable for you, you may find as time passes that your illness interferes less and less in your daily life. In fact, you may realize that you can return to work and resume most of your former activities. In this case too, dependency is no longer an important issue for you.

WHEN DEPENDENCY IS A PROBLEM

Individuals with strong, autonomous natures, however, may have deep problems coming to terms with dependency. They may hate being in an "inferior" position, and despise being pitied. Like Marion, they may become depressed. Or they may feel shame, embarrassment, and/or guilt about needing, asking for, and/or taking help. In fact, rather than showing their appreciation toward their caregivers, they may drive them away with anger. Demanding much of themselves, they often make unrealistic demands of others, thus rendering the task of caregiving difficult and unfulfilling. Indeed, not only will they resent their caregivers, but eventually their caregivers may come to resent them in return.

After quadruple bypass heart surgery, a widower named Harry tried to hang on to every measure of independence he could muster. He often clashed with his son and daughter-in-law, resisting the help he received from them, even though he so desperately needed it. At worst, he never accepted his dependence and incurred his family's anger and resentment at his constant demands and complaints.

"Why should I go out of my way to help Harry anymore?" his daughter-in-law, Deirdre, asked during a family session. "He calls up crying that he needs me to do his grocery shopping for him. I feel sorry for him and go on his errands. But then, instead of thanking me for taking time out of my busy day, he criticizes whatever I bring home for him. I don't have time or energy for this nonsense anymore. I don't care how sick he is." Unfortunately, Harry, as do many fiercely independent individuals, played out his own worst fear—that he would be rejected by those he needs the most.

Another patient, Katie, didn't require hospitalization after her diagnosis of multiple sclerosis, but had such a fear of becoming dependent that she had a nightmare symbolizing it. Katie dreamed that her husband, Bill, was attempting unsuccessfully to push her through a revolving door as she sat in a wheelchair (her fantasy of what might become of her). While he was struggling with the door, she tried desperately to hold on to the hands of their two small children.

The dream depicted Katie's worst fear: if she ever became dependent, Bill would be incapable of handling his new role as caretaker. He would go round and round, unable to find solutions to their family problems.

Katie's fears were based on her realistic evaluation of their personalities. A highly independent individual, she had instinctively married a man who was and would always be dependent on her. But now, facing the possibility of relying physically on her husband at some time in the future, she felt sure that he would become befuddled. Intuitively, she believed that Bill could never cope with her increased demands and would eventually leave her. After much reflection and discussion, she decided to leave him. Given her personality, situation, and age, it was a good decision for her.

If you don't recognize and resolve your fear of dependency, you may discover the destruction that occurs in the vacuum: marriages and families often split without the affected parties ever realizing why. I have seen husbands leave dependent wives, and adult children place parents in nursing homes, feeling it was their only alternative. Most of these people were totally unaware that the resolution of their dependency issues would have saved them much heartache and difficulty.

FINDING A BALANCE

The situations I have just described are extreme and relatively rare. It is uncommon for a mother-in-law and daughter-in-law to fulfill each other's needs for emotional and physical dependency so perfectly. It is equally unusual for a husband to be so emotionally dependent that he cannot manage his chronically ill wife's changing needs.

Most of us find ourselves between these two poles. Sometimes we need to rely on others (and want to make sure we have someone to lean on), and at other times we need to be autonomous and assert ourselves.

Florence, a cancer survivor, told me that she began reasserting her independence as she recovered her strength. "After my diagnosis and surgery and while I was undergoing chemotherapy," she explained, "all I wanted to hear from my husband was 'Don't worry. I'm here for you.' I hungered for every ounce of support I could get. Having Mickey take care of me felt wonderful. But after a while it was important for me to pick up some of my old responsibilities! I wanted to get back to my old self." Nevertheless, Florence wisely recognized that she would always be more physically dependent than she had been before her illness had struck.

The struggle to find a balance between being dependent and independent can be long and trying. It can also be lonely, even if your family and friends do their best to be helpful. If you have difficulty accepting assistance, it may require a major effort on your part to do so. Just remember that how you deal with dependency is uniquely your own process. It cannot be a reflection of how others want you to be—there is no "right" or "wrong" way.

In taking charge, your ultimate goal is to be comfortable with how you deal with being dependent: to accept the physical limitations your disease has placed on you, and to be able to ask for and accept help, while at the same time maintaining your sense of integrity and autonomy.

TAKING STOCK

To help you come to terms with your dependency issues, you must first understand how you feel about being dependent. The following checklist will help you identify your attitudes on this subject.

Thinking back on your life before you became ill, ask your-self the following questions:

- Did I find it difficult to ask others for help?
- Was it easy for me to ask for help?
- Under what circumstances was I willing to accept help?

Now that you are struggling with a long-term illness, ask yourself the following questions:

- Am I finding it difficult to ask others for help?
- Is it easy for me to ask for help?
- Under what circumstances am I willing to accept help?
- How much help do I actually need?
- What can I do for myself?
- In what areas must I rely on others?
- On whom can I rely if I need help?
- How would I feel if they turned me down?
- Do I have a stand-by support group if those who primarily help can't fulfill their duties?
- Do I feel critical or embarrassed if others help me? If so, how do I react?
- How do I react if people offer me help that I don't need or want?

Do you feel differently about dependency now than you did before you became ill? If you do, it is most likely due to your medical condition. You are making a transition from being "well" to being "sick."

You may have always believed that you were, as one of my patients put it, "the toughest cuss in the world." It was frightening for him to realize how dependent on others he actually was—even before his illness. On the other hand, as you answer these questions, you may discover that you've always hated being dependent—your illness didn't create the problem.

Once you identify where you fit on this continuum, you will put yourself back in charge of your life by recognizing and anticipating your fears. You will also be ready to take the next step: making the adjustments necessary to mastering your fear of dependency.

CONQUERING YOUR DEPENDENCY ISSUES

In my years of practice, I have found that people suffering from long-term illnesses can go through several stages as they adjust to their new dependent status. These include:

- Experiencing the grieving process
- Learning to ask for and receive help
- Setting reasonable and reachable goals
- Establishing new goals within a safe framework
- Giving to others
- Working out financial issues
- Becoming involved in medical decisions.

Let's look at these steps in greater detail.

Experiencing the Grieving Process

Just as with identity issues (see chapter 6), it is important for you to grieve your waning independence. Establish what you have lost by writing it down or sharing it with family, friends, clergy, or a therapist. You may have physical limitations that impair your mobility and force you to depend on a wheelchair or walker to get around. You may need others to tend to your physical care. As the result of a stroke, you may have become unable to write or you may have lost strength in an arm or leg. You may no longer be able to drive, shop, or climb stairs. These are all significant losses of independence.

You can counter some deficits with substitutions. For example, Raquel was no longer able to do the family food marketing, but she could still clip coupons, plan meals, and draw up the weekly shopping list. Richard had to give up driving, but he was able to remain the family's vacation planner and chief navigator.

Of course, these substitutions may not seem equal when compared to the originals, and you may feel a deep sadness as you consider them. But your native intelligence will come to your rescue now as you slowly and perhaps painfully realize that you are accepting reality. After all, it is likely that your illness has placed some physical limitations on you. Nevertheless, in this difficult first stage, you will discover your remaining assets, and you will learn what to look forward to.

You may also find it helpful to admit your fears to your loved ones, and thus share with them your grieving process. Depending on your coping style (see chapter 2), you might wish to say, for example, "It's frightening for me to be so dependent now. It is such a great change for me. I know I will make the transition in time, but right now it is scary. I want you to understand my feelings and I appreciate any support you can give me as I make this transition." Statements such as these may diminish your fears and can help you remain in control of your life.

Learning to Ask for and Receive Help

Before you can ask for and receive help, you must first establish whom you can count on in times of difficulty. Who can help you and under which circumstances would you call upon them? (See p. 106 for instructions on how to map out your support network.) Since you know that at some time you will need to appeal to these people for physical or emotional support, you should consider in what manner you feel comfortable doing so. We all find our own ways to ask for and accept help.

If you are the type of person who clings to his independence at the risk of alienating others, like Harry, you might experience great pain in feeling beholden to others to get your needs met. That pain may be translated into an angry outburst as others attempt to help you. It's the wise individual who realizes that he needs his family members. To help yourself, you might say to yourself or your family members "I hate being like this. I'm the father—always the one you could depend on. It's killing me to ask for help, but I know I have to."

What should you do if a friend or loved one offers help that you don't need? A gentle phrase such as "I love you and appreciate your concern, but I need to do this on my own," can inform your caregiver that you want your independence, even while you leave the door open for future offers. You can also say exactly how you'd like to be helped. Be specific. That will eliminate the chance of confusion or doubt.

It is also possible that, like Marion's husband, Larry, your caregiver is unwittingly hindering your progress toward greater independence out of his own sense of concern, control, and protectiveness. It's natural for your family to feel protective toward you. It's hard for loved ones to see you stumble and fall—literally and figuratively.

If this is so in your case, ask yourself how you can reveal to your caregiver, without hurting his feelings, that you need more independence. Examine the alternatives as carefully and as rationally as you can, and help him see your need for autonomy. You can explain to your loved one that sometimes you will take a tumble but that's OK. You will learn to pick yourself up and go on. You might also tell him that you need to do some things for yourself now that you're getting stronger. You could say "Sometimes I'll need your help, but sometimes I won't."

Negotiate with your caregivers if you wish to repay them for all that they are doing for you. If you can trade services, you will feel more equal in the relationship—there are many small ways in which you can reward your helpers. Of course, if you're feeling weak or vulnerable, you may believe that you have little to offer. In fact, you may perceive that you're always on the receiving end. Yet, even Melissa still found a way to reciprocate. Her poems gave her and her husband great pleasure. It was something she could do that he could not.

Of course, there are myriad ways to square accounts with your family. You don't have to be a poet. If you were once the major wage earner in the family, now you can handle the family finances, doing all the paperwork and tax planning. If you were the family cook, you can research new recipes, plan menus, and maintain the food inventory. This can save valuable time and money. You can also become the family ear—the person who asks others how their day went and really listens. Coping with your own problems will most likely give you extra sensitivity to others. In the process, you may discover that your perception that you're not giving much in return for the help you're receiving is merely that—your perception—and not your family's at all.

Setting Reasonable and Reachable Goals

Almost every day, we read newspaper accounts of heroic individuals with severe physical limitations who find their own ways of being independent. Have you ever asked yourself how the legless woman gets into the wheelchair before she plays tennis? Or how the blind boy gets his bat and knows where to stand when he swings at the baseball? The answer is easy: these individuals get help. They set reachable but realistic goals for themselves. They are able to do what they want, giving them a measure of independence, but they also recognize that they can't do it alone.

You may feel that you'd like to become more independent too, but are afraid to try activities that had been too difficult before. Why not set one tangible, time-limited, reachable goal for yourself? In this way, you are setting up boundaries for yourself that will create within you a feeling of confidence. Reachable goals help to project you into the future.

To determine if your goal is appropriate, ask yourself the following questions:

- Is my goal concrete? ("Being happy" doesn't count. "Going to the market myself" does.)
- Is my goal realistic? ("Getting back to the way I used to be" may be impossible.)
- Do I have permanent physical limitations? If so, how can I factor these into my goal setting?
- Will I need someone to help me achieve my goal?
- Have I set a time limit for achieving my goal? (This helps you to organize your time and thoughts.)

You may be feeling so confused, however, that you can't even focus on a single task. It helps to choose a simple activity, such as taking a shower, shaving, or washing your hair on your own. It may seem silly and insignificant, but set the goal anyway. The task itself may be less important than the fact that you have established it in your struggle to move forward. Value and validate even failed attempts. Take pride in the fact that you tried.

Be sure to adjust your goals to your abilities. If you can't take ten steps, take one. Tomorrow you'll try for two, and eventually you'll reach ten. If you decide that you want to read a book, but find that you're having trouble concentrating on any reading matter, read only a chapter. If that's too much, set a goal to read a page, a paragraph, or just a few sentences. Read what makes sense to you. If you lose the train of thought, stop. Tomorrow, you will try again. Even if you don't do much better the following day, in subsequent attempts you may begin to absorb what you've been perusing. Persistence pays off.

One of your goals might be to remain as physically independent as you can. This is so important to some people that they accomplish astounding feats. For example, Lynette learned how to dismantle her electric cart herself, store it in her trunk, drive to her destination, and finally reassemble it, even though she could not walk! She was extremely resourceful in maintaining whatever level of independence she could for as long as she could. And she did it one step and one goal at a time.

Establishing New Goals Within a Safe Framework

Once you have accomplished the first goal, others may follow. Soon, your range of independent activity may expand to more exciting challenges. From walking ten steps, you may begin walking around the block and then the mall. From reading one paragraph, you may be able to handle several books at once.

Indeed, you may believe that you have lost your independence, when in actuality it is only buried under the weight of your medical problems. Setting new goals helps you to reassert yourself and allows your autonomy to reemerge. Since you will be deciding where, when, and how you are becoming independent, you will find yourself once again in charge of your life.

Giving to Others

Giving to those less fortunate than you can also help you feel more independent and useful. You may become involved in a peer support group and provide others with inspiration and practical advice born of experience. Use your skills and experience to be helpful. I know several people who had been lobbyists in Washington, D.C. Once they were stricken with long-term illnesses, they became extremely effective speakers on behalf of medical groups such as the American Heart Association and the American Cancer Society.

It is possible—and deeply satisfying—to use your own problems to promote the good of others. By giving to others, you may reconnect to "old" parts of your self you might have believed were gone.

Working Out Financial Issues

Financial problems can leave you feeling dependent. It is especially difficult for men to relinquish their financial autonomy if they have been groomed all their lives to be the sole support for their families. Despite the many changes in our society, men today still see themselves as the backbone of the family's financial security. It's hard on some men's egos if they must rely on their wives' health insurance. If they cannot take care of their families, it is a devastating blow.

Those individuals who own their own businesses or are professionals may be able to manage their work and time to suit their new needs. They may continue earning their pre-illness salaries. But those who must go on disability or must depend completely on their spouse's income may feel great pain as they relinquish what had always given them a sense of worth.

Nevertheless, there are ways to work out these financial dependency issues. The first step is to recognize that the situation may be devastating to you, even if your spouse works. You may still feel enormous responsibility for the mortgage payments and your children's college educations.

Once you have recognized the situation, you can look for ways to cope with it. From my experience, every family finds its own way according to its skills and resources. For example, you and your family can reevaluate your goals. You may decide to lower your material expectations and determine what is basic to all of you. In addition, if the "man of the house" can't work, he may still be able to provide leadership in solving family problems. Perhaps the family will function more democratically now that the playing field has been evened a bit.

You may try to bring in some money by working at home, part-time, as your energy allows. Jobs such as telephone sales are well suited to individuals who are too ill to leave the home to work. You might help in your spouse's business—say, by taking care of the books or the ordering from home. Or you may come to see your disability insurance payments as your contribution to the family's income. Perhaps helping out in the home or with the children can satisfy your need to make a concrete contribution.

Becoming Involved in Medical Decisions

There is a range of responses to dealing with one's doctor (see chapter 4). Some individuals prefer that their family members do all the talking while others take full control themselves. Think about where you fit on this continuum. How involved are you in making your own medical decisions?

In order to remain more independent, I recommend that you talk to your physician as much as you can. You, better than family members, can explain how you're feeling. Not that you should exclude your loved ones entirely. They can ask questions you won't think of. But by becoming involved in your medical decisions, you are letting your doctor know that you are in charge and that she must consult you about treatment options. If other family members talk to the doctor exclusively, it puts you in a childlike position. Taking charge will help you feel as independent as you want to be.

MARION TAKES CHARGE

Let's return to the story of Marion, the woman who had had a stroke. Marion had to work through many of these stages on her journey to becoming autonomous once more.

When I began meeting with her on an individual basis, Marion was fending for herself for the first time in three years. She had to make me understand her. Larry wasn't there to interpret.

Calling forth some of her old social skills, Marion immediately asked me if I had any trouble deciphering her faltering speech and strange, unnatural-sounding voice.

"In truth, it is hard for me," I admitted. "But if it becomes too difficult, I'll simply ask you to repeat what you've said." I added, "Marion, even though you believe that you have lost two of your major assets, your physical strength and your verbal abilities, you haven't lost the third—your strong ego. You'll never lose that. It will always be available to you."

Feeling reassured, Marion visibly relaxed. In fact, as we worked together over the next several months, she rarely had to repeat anything. Just giving herself permission to speak for herself put her well on her way to becoming independent again.

As I have advised you to do, I helped Marion begin the grieving process. "What were your most gratifying activities before the stroke?" I asked. "What do you miss the most now?"

"There are so many things." She stopped and shook her head. "I loved my former house. Larry and I had designed and built it ourselves. I loved the garden and the nearby woods. I spent so many happy hours there. We used to go to great parties. You wouldn't know it now, but I had lots of interesting friends. I also often wrote and edited material for Larry's business—that was really valuable to him. I really enjoyed talking—sparring with my friends and doing public speaking. Words, both written and spoken and how they were delivered, were always of prime interest to me."

Marion also grieved for her former physical strength, another source of pride. Whenever she spoke of the pleasure she derived from chopping wood, her eyes lit up. Being physically and mentally fit had been basic to Marion's lifelong self-confidence and independence. Now, in one fell swoop, she believed the stroke had robbed her of it all.

In particular, Marion mourned the loss of her old house. It had always symbolized to her involvement, excitement, and meeting new people. "I just don't identify with my neighbors in the retirement community," she said. Clearly, her house had represented youthful vigor to her. In making their hasty move, she and Larry had overlooked their need for psychological adjustment to their new and different life after the stroke. From leading a full and exciting existence, overnight she and Larry were reduced to days of making the rounds at doctors' offices. No wonder she was so depressed.

Our next step was to review Marion's personal support network. For a person so gregarious, this group turned out to be surprisingly small. She relied mostly on Larry and a daughter from her first marriage. Actually, as she spoke, she realized that she was receiving so much support from her husband, there was little need for anyone else to help her. Larry never left her side.

Now we could pursue a goal that Marion would choose for herself. To get her going, we agreed that she needed one that was concrete and realistic. We also agreed that she needed a deadline.

After thinking for a few minutes about her goal, Marion blurted out, "Peace of mind."

"That sounds wonderful," I replied, "but you might choose something a little simpler and less abstract."

"What do you mean?" she asked.

I offered several examples. "How about going to the grocery store tomorrow or unpacking your moving boxes by next Thursday?"

At first these goals sounded almost silly in light of the torment she was experiencing. But after a few minutes, Marion flashed an understanding smile, and I saw that her quick intelligence was still very much with her. She knew exactly what I meant and made plans to shop for some badly needed clothes the following week. We decided that Larry would take her to the store but would leave her alone in the ladies' department. She would handle all of the choosing, trying on, and paying without his intervention.

"Why were you so reluctant to buy new clothes until now?" I asked.

"I was too embarrassed to talk to the saleswomen because of my strange voice," she confessed. "But now I'm ready. I realized that if you could understand and accept these weird sounds coming out of my mouth, certainly a salesperson could too."

The following week, Marion returned and reported her progress. "The saleswoman did have trouble understanding me without Larry's help," she said. "So I felt forced to explain why I talk like I do. I just told her that I had had a stroke. That's all it took! Look, I bought this new sweater and skirt. Aren't they great?"

What a major breakthrough! Not only was Marion asking the saleswoman to accept her, she was also accepting herself. Soon, she moved on to greater challenges. She traveled to an out-of-town family wedding. She began making telephone calls and even invited some friends she'd been out of touch with for dinner. Then she demonstrated to me, and to herself, that she was ready to move on with her life—she unpacked those moving boxes that had been sitting for so long in her forlorn living room.

Once Marion took this step, she resumed many of the activities that had formerly given her so much pleasure. She became involved in community organizations and took up public speaking again. She and Larry joined a club for stroke survivors and almost immediately she became its leader. "I'm speaking at each meeting," she told me excitedly. "I tell others how I overcame my embarrassment at the strange sound of my voice."

I asked Marion and Larry to come together to our last session. He no longer answered the questions that I directed to Marion and could barely contain his joy when she openly and strongly disagreed with him on some points. Perhaps her words did occasionally come out a little slowly, but her thoughts were just as sharp and quick as they had always been.

Although Marion would always be a "patient" and thus dependent on others, she could still retain her wonderful independent spirit. On her own again, Marion learned to cope with real dependency needs: she learned to distinguish what she truly needed from others and what she could do on her own. She was managing her life again.

GOING FORTH

Most likely, dependency was not something you wanted. Your illness imposed it on you. Now, what are you going to do? Your only choice is to cope.

How you overcome your fear of dependency will be unique to you. Follow your instincts, and don't be too hard on yourself. Once you have come to terms with the degree of dependence in your new life, you can integrate these changes so that they feel normal to you. The transition doesn't happen overnight. Give yourself time. Soon, you will evolve from feeling helpless to feeling helpful again, an active member of your family and society.

REMEMBER

- Dependency is an issue for all of us, whether healthy or ill.
- Your family or doctor may expect you to be as independent as possible, but there may be times when you will want to be dependent.
- It's natural to be dependent in the hospital.
- Some people have more problems with dependency than others.
- Accept the physical limitations your condition has placed on you.
- It's best to strive to achieve a balance between independence and dependence.

- If you need help, find a way that's comfortable to ask for and receive it.
- If you don't need help, find a way to assert your autonomy without hurting those who offer aid.

THINGS TO DO

- Take stock.
- Experience the grieving process.
- Learn to ask for and receive help.
- Set reasonable and reachable independence goals.
- Establish new goals within a safe framework.
- Give to others.
- Work out financial issues.
- Become involved in your own medical decisions.
- Try to be as independent as possible.

8.

Mastering Your Fear of Stigma

Stigma, a word originating with the ancient Greeks, once referred to a tattoo that marked slaves and criminals. A person with a stigma was to be avoided, especially in public places. Over the years the term has evolved. Today, it has come to mean a sign of disgrace or degeneration, a stain of reproach or infamy.

The eminent social psychologist Erving Goffman studied this phenomenon in his 1963 book, *Stigma.* He explains that now the word can also refer to a person who is disqualified from social acceptance because an illness has changed his external appearance or behavior. And therein lies the rub.

If your long-term condition has altered how you look or behave, you and your family may have to confront the issue of stigma. Indeed, it has the potential for becoming a major emotional problem, especially since most people don't recognize stigma at first and don't realize how it can affect their lives on a daily basis.

Stigma is not to be underestimated. It can be subtle and insidious. You may find that your coworkers stop asking you to lunch or that friends make social arrangements without you. You will feel the results without understanding the cause.

It's important to distinguish between stigma and a loss of your old self-image (see chapter 6). Self-image refers to your own feelings about yourself, while stigma refers to the responses of others to you.

In coping with your long-term illness, you may have become quite comfortable with the way you feel about yourself. You may no longer perceive yourself as "damaged goods." You may even feel terrific! Your new self-image is intact.

But no matter how well you have integrated your new persona, society may respond to you differently. People may avoid you or may stop and stare. Children may point at you and ask loudly, "Why does that lady have only one leg?" You may see strangers shake their heads and whisper before averting their gaze, or you may hear teenagers giggling behind your back.

These reactions are painful to experience. The bias against those who are disabled or disfigured is as old as mankind itself. It is a reflection of our inherent fear of the unknown and our vulnerability. We are frightened of those who are different from ourselves.

These prejudices may have little to do with you personally, but if you do not address them, they can haunt you and your family for the rest of your life.

STIGMA CAN HURT YOU

Stigma can cause you and your loved ones deep personal pain. Every time you are introduced to new people, they may see you as "flawed." They will never know you as you once were—healthy and whole. Every time you see old friends, you may find they no longer treat you as they once did. They may speak to you cautiously, act as if they're walking on eggshells, or even refer to you in the third person, as if you weren't really there. You may try to dismiss their behavior, believing that it's their problem, not yours. Nevertheless, you cannot completely avoid it.

You may become hurt, angry, and/or impatient at what you perceive as insensitivity, cruelty, and/or unfairness. You may feel frustrated and impotent at confronting all of mankind. You can't do anything about the bias. You wonder, "Isn't it enough to cope with the physical problems? Now this?" You didn't choose to become disfigured; your illness imposed it.

As you rail against the inequities and the indignities you must endure, others may increasingly view you as hostile. You feel "they" are insensitive and cruel—"they" don't understand you. You feel sorry for yourself; you're a victim. You sense that your family is ashamed of you, and you discover that they have been hiding their humiliation in subtle ways. You begin to take the slights personally, even though you know your illness is the real cause. Yet if you show your anger, others may feel that you are releasing your frustrations on them. You may even buy into the stigma and come to believe that you are an "outsider" and a blemished person.

GOING INTO HIDING

If the outward manifestations of your illness are immediately apparent (as in a physical injury or a debilitating stroke), you have no choice but to deal with them straightaway. On the other hand, if your illness progresses slowly, you may have been able to conceal its symptoms and thus avoid dealing with stigma—for a while, anyway. But, keeping your condition a secret can prove destructive to you and your loved ones. I treated two young men who left their wives upon learning that the women knew of their illness before marriage. The husbands weren't angry at their wives for being sick. They were angry at being deceived.

Nevertheless, you may believe that as long as you can hide your bare head under a wig, your swollen arm within a long sleeve, your scarred leg inside your trousers, you can put off coping with this ugly issue. However, when the stumbling becomes obvious, the eyelids droop more heavily, or the cane must be traded for a wheelchair, you have little alternative but to confront the unpleasant side of society. When you must make a major change in your behavior, after hiding your symptoms for years, you are forced to come to terms with the way human beings treat someone who looks or acts different.

Indeed, crisis may occur when you can no longer cover up the outward manifestations of the disease. You may decide that being up against the world is just too overwhelming. You may even choose to withdraw from society under these circumstances. You may become a shut-in, depriving yourself and your loved ones of contact with friends or other constructive outlets. The illness becomes a deep, dark secret.

Yet the hurt, anger, and hostility that this response engenders can increase stress for you as well as your family. When you withdraw from society, you limit human contact. Since you have chosen this position, your family may become angry at you for having denied them their freedom.

I have a profound personal familiarity with the issue of stigma and hiding. As a parent, I experienced all of these problems and reactions with my daughter. It took me two years to realize that I could not and should not hide Linda's heart condition from the world.

When she was an infant, I had little difficulty conceal-ing her ailment. Lying in her crib or carriage, she didn't exert herself. The oxygen deprivation caused by her heart defects never became apparent. However, once she began walking and running after her little friends in the neigh-borhood park, I could no longer hide her infirmity. When-ever she exerted herself, her lips and fingertips turned blue. Whenever she really became tired, she instinctively stopped running and crouched to help alleviate the spell.

I didn't want any of the other mothers at the park to wit-ness my child's color change. It showed that she was ill. But, more important, I couldn't bear for anyone to see her crouch. This made her seem odd and different. It also made me feel odd and different. I feared that people would ask questions I neither wanted nor knew how to answer.

Therefore, just as Linda's lips began changing colors—before it became obvious to others or the oxygen depriva-tion was bad enough to cause her to crouch—I would scoop her up in my arms. Keeping my eyes on her face to monitor her color, I placed her in her stroller, and as quickly as I could, ran down the street, shouting some excuse over my shoulder to the other mothers as I retreated.

I really never thought about my actions until they became a regular occurrence. But when, time after time, I had to face my child as we were leaving the park, I began to feel guilty about my behavior. "What am I doing?" I asked myself. "Am I hiding this innocent child?" As I realized that I was, I began to cry in shame. But I also decided that I could not do this for the rest of her life. Mulling it over, I concluded that if I continued to run and hide "our" prob-lem, I might face a mental breakdown myself.

I knew that I had to come to grips with my fear of stigma to release us from the self-imposed exile I was creating.

COMING OUT OF HIDING

If you feel, as I did, that staying out of sight is too destructive, that you can no longer tolerate avoiding others, and that you would rather risk the hurt than isolate yourself forever, then you can confront the stigma realistically, no matter how distasteful or difficult it may be.

Chances are, the catalyst for change may occur once you decide you can no longer hide or lie about your symptoms. Indeed, you may feel that you can't live in fear of being found out anymore. You may be engulfed by anxiety, worrying:

- "Have my coworkers noticed any changes in my behavior?"
- "I lied about my physical condition on the new job application. I've never lied before. Will someone expose me?"
- "Will my colleagues observe that I've parked in the handicapped spot? Will they report this to the boss?"

You may also worry about your friends:

- "Have they observed that I'm eating with my left hand instead of my right?"
- "Are they aware that I go home from parties earlier?"
- "Can they detect that my glasses are getting thicker?"
- "Do they notice that I never play tennis anymore?"
- "Do they see that I refuse desserts now?"

The stress of remaining silent becomes unbearable. The consequences of withholding the truth may be worse than exposing your flaws to the world. You fear a mental breakdown or the disintegration of your marriage. Either of these, you decide, would be worse than telling. You see yourself as a stranger, even to yourself. You have reached the point of no return. You want to stop running; you're tired of being depressed; you know your family is suffering. As your physical symptoms worsen, you fear your anxiety will aggravate your condition. Coming out of hiding becomes a matter of personal survival.

One way or another, right or wrong, clumsy, painful, and embarrassing or not, you must figure out a way to cope with the ongoing stigma. You have realized that it is impossible to change mankind. Yet you have also come to the conclusion that you must get on with your life. Once you have resolved not to be intimidated or frightened by an anticipated or real response of insensitivity, you will have to decide what to do. You can't control others' prejudices, but you can control how you deal with them.

TAKING CHARGE OF STIGMA

You have it in your power to handle stigma. You are right; you cannot change the world's view of you, but since you realistically recognize what you cannot do, you can also realistically recognize what you can do. *Dealing with all of society may be too much, but you can deal with one person at a time.* You are capable of changing how you cope with one person's insensitive questions or how you respond to hurts or slights aimed at your odd-looking leg, not you. You don't need to be a victim of stigma. You can take charge of your life again.

In order to overcome your fear of stigma, you may wish to follow these steps:

- Look at the world realistically.
- Reveal your secret.

- Rehearse.
- Use a support group.
- Include the family.
- Don't take slights personally.
- Take control of how you present yourself.
- Take action if you must.

We will cover these steps in greater detail in the remainder of this chapter. But first, I want you to consider people such as Itzhak Perlman, the world-famous concert violinist who wears heavy leg braces, or singer Ray Charles, who is blind. How can they be so comfortable with their disabilities? Why doesn't stigma bother them?

They, like my daughter, grew up with their disabilities and became acclimated to them gradually. As children, they learned how to cope with society's view of someone who is handicapped. Their adult lives and their place in society were not suddenly altered, as yours might be.

Indeed, Perlman jokes with his audience about the noise his leg braces make on the wooden stage floor. Ray Charles performed in a TV commercial touting the advantages his blindness gave him over someone who is sighted. Even my daughter was able to tell her friends how far she could walk and to give them permission to go on without her, if she slowed down. These people had become so comfortable with their disabilities that they were able to place those around them at ease. Although each of us makes his or her own decision about how to cope with stigma, it is my hope that the suggestions I present in this chapter will help you achieve this kind of peace.

Look at the World Realistically

You must accept that people are uncomfortable with those who look and act different than the norm. Don't expect the outside world to be warm, sympathetic, or supportive. One person, yes, but all of society? Don't count on it. If you recognize stigma as a given, you won't be as hurt or disappointed in your fellow human beings. Besides, you can't be angry at the whole world. Make the decision not to be intimidated by an anticipated or real insensitive response.

Perhaps the best way to achieve this understanding is to ask yourself how you had reacted to a disabled individual before your illness. Were you put off? Horrified? Did you stare or look away? If all of your life you had been upset by others' afflictions, you may feel even more devastated about your own. For, in truth, you are likely to assume that those around you are reacting to you in the same way that you had reacted to others. (They may or they may not be, however.)

Once you are comfortable with yourself, and acknowledge that others feel squeamish around someone who looks or acts different, you will create your own unique way of revealing your secret. In fact, depending on how visible your symptoms are, you can decide whether you will or will not reveal the truth and to whom.

Reveal Your Secret

You may find it easier to tell a stranger first about your malady, since strangers have no emotional involvement in you or the illness. Or you may tell a close family member if you feel the relative will continue to love and accept you, no matter what you reveal. It's up to you to determine whom to tell, when to tell it, and what to say. You are in control of this process.

When I vowed to come out of hiding with Linda's problem, I knew that I had to figure out a way to inform others. I decided to tell a complete stranger first. I would see how that emotionally uninvolved individual accepted the idea and my child. I reasoned that if this person could tolerate the terrible news, I would be able to tell others. It would be a test, but I was ready. I didn't know whom I would tell or when, but I was committed to disclosing what had become my deep, dark secret.

As Linda's doctors had directed us, we took her to Florida for the winter; the cold air in Washington, D.C., was too difficult for her to breathe. One beautiful, sunny February day we found ourselves walking home from the beach. On the way, we stopped at an inviting open-air orange juice stand. The canopy offered some shade from the burning sun, and the countertop was a perfect place for my daughter to rest. I had already observed the color change in her lips; she was getting tired.

I plopped Linda on the counter and ordered two glasses of juice. The vendor said to me, "Look, missus. Your little girl's lips are blue. Maybe she spent too much time in the ocean, eh?"

From the moment this man began speaking, I knew this was the opportunity I had been waiting for. I heard my voice quiver as I responded, "Her lips aren't blue because she's cold. She has a heart condition."

He was silent. But on his face, I could read the question "How could this pretty, innocent child smiling at me have a heart condition?"

After we finished our drinks and I slowly lowered Linda to the sidewalk, we continued on our way home. Holding my daughter's hand in mine, I felt a great sense of calm. The man had survived the "terrible" news, and I had overcome my fear of revealing it. I was also relieved of my guilt. I would no longer injure my daughter by hiding her condition from others. It was up to me to choose whom I would tell, when, and where. I had conquered my fear of stigma and was no longer its victim. I had taken charge of my life.

Rehearse

To feel in charge of the conversation, it's important to anticipate what will be said and consider various possibilities. Rehearse your revelation and anticipate possible questions, both sensitive and insensitive.

You can practice your spiel with a willing friend, a therapist, or a member of the clergy. (It might be difficult for family members to remain detached, especially if you ask them to hit you with hard questions and responses.) Try role-playing, in which the trusted individual asks you questions he imagines others would like answered. Tell him not to hold back. You can even write out your words in a journal or speak your confession into a tape recorder. Support groups are also helpful in this regard. The idea is to minimize, as much as possible, the pain of revealing your condition. This is best achieved in a safe place before the fact. (See pp. 175–176 for an example of role-playing.)

Use a Support Group

Sharing a stigma with others in the same situation helps you feel less different—more normal. You will feel that you're not alone. In fact, during a support group for epilepsy patients that I led some years ago, the most common response after the first session was "Gee, there are people who are struggling with the same problems as I am."

A peer support group is also an excellent environment to test your ability to reveal your secret. The group members are strangers who have no emotional involvement with you at first. But they also can understand your feelings and situation in ways that even your most beloved family members may not.

Include the Family

Your family may also feel the stigma and shame of your illness. Indeed, they may experience these emotions even if you don't! I felt shame at Linda's symptoms—to me, the imperfections in her heart indicated some blight on our family. But Linda had no such reaction. If this is the case in your family, you must explain to your loved ones that despite their embarrassment, you've come to feel comfortable with your situation.

Mark had a hard time dealing with his wife's disabilities caused by severe arthritis. One day in my office, he said, "Pushing Allison in a wheelchair feels to me like pushing a stroller—something I had never done in my life. My wife is a curiosity."

Their daughter, Helen, felt equally uncomfortable. "It has bothered me to watch Mom go through the various stages of her disability: first the stumbling, then using one cane, and two. Now the electric cart and the wheelchair."

But Allison's determination to live her life as normally as possible was stronger than her shame and embarrassment. She was able to say to her family, "I know you don't like it, but I'd rather use the cart than stop us from going places. I hold my head up and plow through. I don't care if people look. This is the only way for me to get out. That's the way it is, and I can't change it."

Allison handled her feelings directly and openly. Taking her lead, her family overcame their own humiliation. If she could handle it, they figured, so could they!

Don't Take Slights Personally

If you feel hurt that someone you care about is avoiding you, you can feel angry, but you can also understand that it is not personal. The reaction is a sign of your friend's fear of being different.

If you run into someone who is unpleasant or seems uncomfortable around you, remind yourself that the negative feedback is outside of yourself. You can say to yourself, "I can't control Joan's behavior. It has to do with her fears, not with me. But I can control how I deal with it. I can even anticipate it, so I don't have to be scared or caught off guard." Preparation puts you in control.

Understanding that stigma is a given in many situations, you may choose to:

- Ignore the disparagement.
- Make fun of the situation or laugh yourself.
- Respond in an educational way. (For example, you can say matter-of-factly "I walk with a limp and a cane because the bones in my hip are degenerating.")

It takes courage to face a look of pity or a gesture of avoidance, but separating another's response from their feelings about you—and your own feelings about yourself—will help you to take charge of your life. Your desire to be an active member of society may be stronger than your fear of stigma—and that works to your advantage.

Take Control of How You Present Yourself

Although you may look or sound strange and make others uncomfortable, how you comport yourself does make a difference. For example, if you suffer from a lack of bladder control and have an accident, either you can try to hide your wet clothes or you can hold your head up until they dry. Renee told her teenage daughter that an incontinence problem was not going to stop her from shopping. "I know you don't like it," she said, "but I maintain my composure and go out anyway. What choice do I have?"

George, a Parkinson's patient, handled his stigma issues perfectly by telling his guests, "It's OK. I will be shaking for a few minutes, but don't get frightened. I won't fall." By bringing his problem into the open, he had learned to make others comfortable. Perhaps more important, George had also given himself permission to continue shaking and not feel bad about it.

Sitting in a wheelchair places you at a disadvantage, but here too you can present a positive image. Although you're lower than people who are standing, you can learn to project your voice. Make sure that your hair and clothes are attractive and smile at anyone who might be staring at you. If you project a positive image, others will respond warmly.

You can draw attention to your problem yourself, if you so choose. One of my heart patients, Jackie, receiving physical therapy for injuries sustained in a car accident, revealed how she dealt with a number of "port wine stains" on a leg. When the physiotherapist casually asked what they were, Jackie reported to me that she replied, "Oh, they're birthmarks. Aren't they ugly?" Clearly she wasn't hiding or avoiding questions about them.

In the same spirit, you can choose, as some people do, to make your condition even more visible. A woman who lost her leg to diabetes decorated her crutch, almost inviting people to ask her about her illness. Blessedly—and after far too long—society's attitudes have changed in recent years. Today people ride in the streets in their motorized wheelchairs and remove their prostheses at the beach before taking a plunge. Once you have desensitized yourself, others' comments or stares will no longer be stressful.

Each of us makes his or her own decisions about how we cope with stigma. (You may even grow to appreciate the extra attention you get from having a disability.) Just bear in mind that being respectful of others' feelings puts you in the position of being in charge. Those with whom you come in contact will appreciate your sensitivity and respond in kind. Besides, you can wear your illness as a badge of shame, a badge of courage, or simply a badge of life. It's up to you.

Take Action If You Must

If you feel that stigma shades into prejudice and outright discrimination, contact your local branch of the national health organization dealing with your disease. The society will have volunteers and professionals who are knowledgeable and experienced in dealing with these legal matters. You need not feel victimized.

TODD REVEALS A SECRET

When he first walked into my office, I found Todd to be a handsome, macho sort of guy. He had a beautiful smile, and looked me right in the eye when he spoke to me. He was successful in his work as an engineer in Arlington, Virginia, which required him to do a fair amount of traveling. His wife, Kelly, was bright and pretty. She had only recently begun working part-time. Todd adored their ten-year-old, Steve.

Todd had many friends, especially former schoolmates. They got together weekly to play volleyball in the winter, baseball in the summer, and touch football in the fall. Todd's natural athleticism provided him with a great deal of pride and gratification, since it was a source of recognition among his male friends who were so important in his life.

When Todd first came to see me, however, he and Kelly were seriously depressed. Todd had had MS for nine years, but it never showed. He continued to work, travel, and lead a normal life. He even maintained his athletic schedule every weekend with his old friends. Because his condition was invisible, he had never told anyone about it, not even his parents and in-laws (who lived in distant states) or his son. The only other individual who knew was Kelly, and she was sworn to secrecy.

Yet Todd's neurologist was worried about his mental health. The problem was that his physical symptoms were now becoming more obvious and he could no longer hide them. So, rather than going to lunch with his coworkers, he ate a sandwich at his desk. When asked why he wasn't joining the group as usual, he offered lame excuses. He couldn't bear to tell his colleagues that he had MS, which caused him to stumble over the street curbs he'd need to cross to get to their favorite restaurant. He was behaving differently, and he knew his associates were wondering what was wrong with him.

In addition, Todd had begun to miss his weekend volleyball games. Again, he offered weak explanations of his new behavior: He had to finish some chores around the house; he needed to do some reading. This was atypical for Todd, since he was always a gregarious fellow.

By the time I saw him, this young man knew he had serious problems that he didn't know how to handle. His sources of good feelings about himself were now gravely threatened. It was possible that he would lose them altogether. He watched the process occur slowly. As we discussed his problems, Todd realized that he needed help because he saw no way out.

Todd's loving family and friends were a great potential source of personal support. However, unless these individuals knew of his physical problems, they couldn't help. And Todd had been unwilling to share his secret because he feared that if they discovered he was "different," they would no longer love him.

Moreover, Todd's athleticism and machismo caused him to struggle with his problem alone. He wanted to be one of the guys. He feared being banished from the group in which he had always been the leader. He loved being a jock but now he feared his friends would no longer see him that way.

Todd needed to find a way to begin talking about his illness. In order to do so, he had to understand his fears: what was rational and what was not. Did he really think that because he couldn't walk straight or play ball his lifelong friends would reject or avoid him? Were his good looks and high energy the only reasons they cared about him? Wasn't there something else about him that was lovable and attractive?

I didn't have to work very hard to help Todd recognize that these fears were unfounded. He was secure in his awareness that these people loved him. He just couldn't bear for them to see him as being "flawed."

He sensed the discomfort of strangers in the airport. Those who saw him sway seemed to avoid him. "Were they afraid of coming close to me?" he wondered. "Were they talking behind my back?" He had always been so well liked, an insider. "Am I now being forced to look at the world from the outside in?" he asked.

As we talked, Todd realized how important it was for him to be himself. Hiding and avoiding were unnatural to him. They even drained valuable physical energy. Todd's goal was easy to target but difficult to accomplish: he needed to open up and tell his secret, but when and to whom?

"Which person in your life do you want to tell first?" I asked him.

Todd's reply came quickly and without hesitation. "I want to tell Steve," he said. "Later I'll tell my parents, and then everyone else. For now, he's the most important person in my life. He'll be the hardest to tell, but I won't do it until I'm completely ready." He was resolved.

In the following sessions, Todd and I methodically prepared for his fateful moment with his son. He began rehearsing his message in my office. This allowed him to practice and gave him the chance to experience revealing the truth. He could feel the sting that accompanied his painful first admission in a safe place where we could manage his feelings.

I was to take Steve's part in a role-playing session, asking every question I believed he might pose. I warned Todd that I might ask scary and difficult questions—some that Steve might not think of. But Todd was ready. He knew what to expect from me. Nonetheless, he broached the subject with much difficulty.

"Honey," he began, "I have something to tell you. Maybe it's something you've already wondered about. Do you remember last week, when you heard me tell Marvin that I couldn't play volleyball? You asked me why I wasn't going and I told you that I had to fix the garage door. You had a funny look on your face, and you were right. I would have preferred playing with my friends to fixing something around the house, but to tell you the truth, I really can't play anymore. It's not that I don't love it. I do! I just have a physical problem that prevents me from playing."

Tears rolled down Todd's cheeks as he spoke. In the privacy of my office, he didn't have to fight them.

I responded as Steve might. "What kind of physical problem? Is it serious?"

As an aside, Todd asked me, "How do I explain MS?"

"Just keep going," I reassured him. "Say it as it comes."

"Well," he said, "I have a disease called multiple sclerosis and I will have it all my life. I found out about it ten years ago, right after you were born, but it never bothered me until recently. It's a funny disease. It comes and goes. Sometimes I feel better and sometimes worse. I never know how I'll feel. Until last year, except for some tingling in my hands and feet, I hardly knew I had it. Now, and I guess you've noticed, sometimes I fall and sometimes I'm very tired."

There. He had done it. But I pressed on. "How much worse is it going to get?" I asked. "Are you going to die?" I felt this to be Steve's chief concern, and Todd was ready for the question.

Without hesitation he responded, "Yes, I'm going to die someday, but probably not for a long time and probably not from MS. The worst thing that may happen is that I might end up in a wheelchair." As Todd spoke these last, difficult words, he looked me directly in the eye. Now, with his hands visibly shaking, he asked, "Will you still love me?" That was his primary fear.

"Yes, Daddy," I said, basing my answer on what I thought Steve would say, given Todd's description of him and their relationship. "I will always love you, no matter what happens to you. It doesn't matter to me if you play basketball or sit in a wheelchair."

Todd watched my face carefully. When I finished, he was silent. His trembling had subsided and the tears had dried on his face. After a few minutes, he said, very calmly, "I think I'm ready. I'll take him on a picnic this week and let you know what happened."

Todd came into his next session looking inches taller and sporting a wide grin. Before he related the details of his encounter, he told me how good it felt to have the tremendous weight of his problems off his shoulders. Since his conversation with Steve, he had felt a surge of energy he no longer thought possible. "Steve's response to my confession wasn't much different than the way we had rehearsed it," he confided. "He had already suspected something. Now it all made sense to him."

Having revealed his secret to his son, Todd felt ready to share it with others, in much the same order we had laid out earlier. Although we rehearsed for these meetings, they seemed much easier because the ice was already broken.

As Todd completed each one, he reported that, when compared to the first, they were a breeze. During each meeting, he learned that even though he was "different," his friends and loved ones still felt the same about him. He might have changed on the outside, but he remained the same person on the inside. Indeed, he learned that he could manage any new encounters now. Like me, he could tell whomever he wanted, whatever he wanted, whenever he wanted. Todd had overcome his fear and was back in charge of his life!

REMEMBER

- If your illness affects the way you look or behave, you might have to deal with stigma.
- Distinguish between stigma and a loss of self-image. The former is external while the latter is internal.
- It's natural for people to avoid those who look or act differently. They are frightened.
- Crisis can occur when you can no longer conceal your affliction, especially if you believe that you must.
- If you go into hiding, you may become a shut-in.
- The stress of obfuscating the truth can become unbearable.
- You can't change all of society, but you can deal with one person at a time.

THINGS TO DO

- Look at the world realistically.
- Ask yourself how you dealt with others' disabilities before you became ill.
- Reveal your secret to a stranger or friend.

- Rehearse with a safe but detached individual.
- Use a support group.
- Include the family.
- Don't take slights personally.
- Ignore any disparagements.
- Make fun of the situation or laugh at yourself.
- Respond in an educational way.
- Take control of how you present yourself.
- Wear your illness like a badge of courage. It is.

9.

Mastering Your Fear of Abandonment

Heoward, a young physician, his mother, Gladys, and his wife, Bonnie, were referred to me because they were struggling with the consequences of placing Gladys in a small nursing home. Despite her diagnosis of Alzheimer's, Gladys had been living with them for several years. Her situation had been manageable until recently, when she began wandering unattended from the house. Howard and Bonnie were deeply concerned that Gladys might become lost or injured. Their young children often ran out and followed their grandmother down the street, creating a dangerous situation for all. Yet Howard and Bonnie feared hurting Gladys's feelings by discussing alternatives to home-care with her. They made the move without bringing up these difficult issues.

This couple felt extremely guilty about turning Gladys's care over to "strangers." Howard had been an only child—the apple of his mother's eye. He owed his medical education to her efforts. But there was no way he could provide the twenty-four-hour-a-day supervision that his mother increasingly required. While he believed that by giving up the reins to someone else he was abandoning Gladys, he saw no alternative. He researched and placed her in the best facility he could find: an intimate, homelike setting in which he believed she would be comfortable and well cared for.

Gladys was furious. She believed that her family had let her down. The move was made without her consent, causing recriminations, ill will, and anger all around. "Is this my repayment for all of my years of sacrifice?" she asked angrily. Beneath it all she felt frightened and abandoned. "Now that I'm sick and disabled, my son left me all alone," she later wept. "He must not love me anymore. He doesn't even want me in his home." In her confusion and rage, Gladys was crying out for help. Her fear of abandonment had blinded her to the real issues that she and her family faced.

FEAR OF ABANDONMENT IS BASIC TO ALL OF US

Everyone experiences the fear of abandonment at one time or another in life. Abandonment may be one of our greatest fears—sometimes it's even more powerful than the fear of death. It is a most primitive and terrifying emotion, harking back to infancy, when a mother's withdrawal literally jeopardizes a baby's survival.

With the advent of a long-term illness, this fear is exacerbated, especially if one is feeling weak or helpless. In fact, now that you have a chronic condition, you may find that you sometimes "feel like a baby": you want to be coddled and cared for; you are helpless; you crave the same unconditional, secure love you received from your parents. But even while you want it, you also know that you are an adult. You recognize that you can never get such complete and total acceptance again—not even from your spouse or closest family.

You realize there are limits to what your loved ones will tolerate, yet you don't know what they are. *The fear of abandonment is closely linked to your testing your family's limits.* It is impossible for family members to completely meet your every need. When you fear abandonment, you may push at their limits to reassure yourself continually that they love you. Underlying the testing behavior is a deeper fear that your loved ones will leave, never to return, because of complaints, exhaustion, the inability to manage, or a desire to escape.

Once you recognize that this dynamic exists, you will have the option to do something about it—to take charge.

THE MANY FACES OF ABANDONMENT

You will never experience fear of abandonment in isolation (as you might suffer loss of control or self-image). Abandonment exists in relation to others, so your fear may manifest itself in conflicts with loved ones. You want love, caring, and attention, but somehow you're not quite getting the kind of assurance from family or friends that would make you feel secure. The following situations have made a number of my patients feel as if they were being abandoned (even if they weren't):

- Just yesterday, your wife told you that she could manage, but today you hear her crying in the next room. You wonder, "Is she really able to handle me now?"
- Your sister didn't call today, as she usually does. Although she always asks, "How do you feel?" does today's silence mean that she's really tired of hearing your complaints?

- You're waiting for your daughter to pick you up for a doctor's appointment, and she's fifteen minutes late. She's never late! Does this mean that she "forgot" the time?
- You don't mind that your husband wants to play cards once a week with his friends, but now he's planning a weekend fishing trip. Does this mean that he'd rather spend time with his friends than you?
- Your wife works three days a week, but now she wants to take evening courses. Does this mean that she's tired of being at home with you?
- Your husband began sleeping in your young son's bed two weeks ago, but hasn't returned to your bed. Does that mean he will never come back?

In all of these cases, my patients felt frightened and needed reassurance from their loved ones.

ABANDONMENT CAN BE CONFUSING

Fear of abandonment is a complex emotion. It can give rise to many confusing, conflicting, and ambivalent feelings for you and your family. For example, you worry that your family is tired and frustrated. They stay home with you night after night because you cannot get out, and you wonder if they feel bored or resentful. You urge them to take some time for themselves, but when they do, you believe they can't wait to get away from you. You fear that you are the cause of their exhaustion and that they're tired of the burden. It's a no-win situation.

So, you try to read their minds: they must be angry at you because you insisted on taking a family trip knowing that it would be difficult for you to maneuver. You suspect they're resentful because you begged them to stay home from an event they really wanted to attend, but you were feeling particularly lonely. Unfortunately, now you feel lonelier still, since you believe they're angry at you for making them stay.

You realize that you're only guessing at how your family feels. You really want to know the truth, so you ask. But you get a partial answer that's only partially satisfying. "What's the point of talking about something I can't do anything about?" sums up your spouse's frustration, which doesn't move you nearer your goal of feeling safe and secure. (This answer, by the way, is more typical of men, who believe that they should solve problems actively; women are more likely to believe they can resolve a situation by simply talking about it.)

If you press further, however, you may get a result you don't want: avoidance, increased misunderstanding, or even hostility. You and your spouse may have divergent agendas. Whereas you feel neglected, your spouse may feel put upon; while you're seeking reassurance, she may be needing respite.

WHY IT'S HARD TO TALK ABOUT YOUR FEARS

It's difficult to air such deep-seated, childlike fears when you're feeling vulnerable and weak. Besides, your family may have problems discussing your fears because they too are feeling confused and conflicted. Their guilt may keep them from revealing their true feelings. Because you are the sick one, they may feel they are not entitled to complain (see chapter 3).

Moreover, you may believe that somehow you are undeserving of your family's care: sometimes you're unlovable, even mean, ornery, and difficult to be with. You may feel that you are an added burden to your loved ones—maybe you're not worth bothering about. You may be torn between wanting to hear the truth and wanting only reassurance.

ARE THEY REALLY ABANDONING YOU?

In order to begin coping with this complex fear, it may help to understand what the word *abandonment* actually means. Several of my patients believed they were being abandoned. But on examining their predicament carefully, they came to see that they weren't.

The unabridged edition of *The Random House Dictionary of the English Language* defines abandonment as "to forsake utterly." From my experience, I can assert that in the case of long-term illnesses, that usually doesn't occur. An individual may leave (she may retreat from a situation with which she can no longer cope) but she usually returns—she does not break the connection.

Look at Howard and Gladys's case. Once he had placed his mother in the nursing home, he visited her every morning and evening. Using his physician's prerogative, he checked her medical charts daily. In truth, he hadn't abandoned his mother at all; he had done and continued to do everything he could for her. When he came to that realization, he felt it necessary to explain his actions to her. He told Gladys, "I love you and will always be there for you. I've moved you here because you need round-the-clock care. I was frightened that you would get hurt or lost if you stayed with us. And, I was afraid I would hurt your feelings by talking to you about it."

Gladys finally understood her son's motives. Howard had placed her in the nursing home out of caring and concern for her safety—not because he no longer wished to have her in his house.

However, until Gladys felt reassured of her son's continuing devotion, her fears intensified. She had worried that she would be left all alone in the world and that she would die, forsaken and miserable.

You too may feel this way at times. But it's important to recognize that this fear is exaggerated. It may be brought on by your anxiety. Nevertheless, it magnifies all of the issues you must deal with. In order to take charge, you must sort out "real" abandonment from the "imagined" variety.

Some of my patients have tested their families by shouting at them "All right, then, why don't you put me in a nursing home?" By exhibiting this sort of behavior, my patients were seeking reassurance. Most often they got the desired response: "No, you know I'd never do that."

On the other hand, it is also true that some family members actually do leave without intending to return, either literally or figuratively. These people can no longer tolerate what they feel is an untenable situation. The husband who, night after night, comes home from work (slaving to pay the medical bills) to find a wife berating him mercilessly for being late, or the wife who is doing everything to keep her husband comfortable, only to hear him constantly denigrate her management skills, may feel that he or she has reached the limits of their endurance.

Although your whole family might feel frightened about talking about this fear, it is vital to do so. Even though the subject of abandonment is very painful, it must be broached. You may feel afraid and guilty, as may your loved ones, but your very survival may hinge on your being able to focus on this difficult issue. After all, you are dependent on your loved ones for your care. If misunderstandings continue or escalate, you or your family may take actions (such as separation, divorce, or institutionalization) out of fear or guilt that you all might regret later.

Before you conquer your fear, you must confront it. Consider the following difficult situations that arose in two families who had come to see me for help. In the first case, Greg and Susan were unable to come to terms with their abandonment issues until it was almost too late. In the second, Joe and Amanda found a way out of their morass before they had to resort to the drastic measures they'd considered—divorce and even suicide.

THE IMPORTANCE OF TAKING PART IN A DECISION

Three years before Greg and Susan came to see me, Susan had been diagnosed with multiple sclerosis (MS). Despite the fact that this couple had sought the best care available in the country, the disease had progressed furiously. Now, at the age of fifty, Susan had deteriorated from being a university history professor, active mother of four, and capable athlete to being a complete invalid: she could move only her eyelids. She communicated by blinking and shifting her eyes in response to an alphabet chart and by using a specially rigged computer.

During this difficult period, Greg gave his wife the best home care he could. This was easy for him, since he loved and respected her deeply. At first, he cared for Susan alone. But when the task grew too difficult, he hired a day nurse, managing her night care himself.

When Susan's physical condition declined to the point that she was no longer able to breathe on her own, she made the difficult decision of continuing on a respirator. The alternative was certain death.

Although Susan had chosen life, she and Greg had very different ideas about her actual living arrangements after she had been connected to the ventilator. Susan assumed she would return home with her equipment after her hospital stay. But Greg had arranged for her to go directly into a nursing home.

This inconsistency in expectations occurred because neither Susan nor Greg had been capable of talking about the future with the other. These two exceptionally bright, articulate individuals, who had always been able to work out any problems they had encountered, were now totally crippled by their emotions.

When I asked Susan if they had discussed her future, she said they had, but I knew Greg had never made his feelings clear. Perhaps Susan was unable to hear what her husband was saying; perhaps Greg was unable to say what his wife needed to hear. Whatever the reason, Susan felt abandoned and betrayed by the person closest to her. Greg was disappointed at what he felt was Susan's insensitivity to him and their children.

Although Susan felt that her husband had abandoned her, in truth her situation was much like Gladys's. Greg visited the nursing home every evening after work and brought their children on the weekends. He talked to her nurses daily and even took a job he didn't enjoy to cover her nursing home expenses. Greg had not abandoned his wife. He and their children loved Susan very much; they just could no longer provide at home the complex care she required.

Had this couple been able to discuss all of the ramifications of Susan's life on a respirator, they might have found a solution to their dilemma that would have included home care (such as temporary respite for Greg or a small addition to the house for a live-in nurse). Unfortunately, by the time I was consulted, too much anger had passed between them and their extended families. Eventually, the best that could be done to alleviate a volatile situation was for Susan to move into her own apartment with twenty-four-hour-a-day nursing care. Greg continued to visit and care for her there for four more years until she died.

Before that, Susan came to see that Greg loved her too much ever to abandon her. Sadly, this realization came too late to stave off the intense emotional pain both had suffered. Had they been able to face and deal with their abandonment issues earlier, perhaps many of these difficulties would have been avoided.

TESTING THE LIMITS OF LOYALTY

By the time Abe's kidney specialist had referred him to me, his kidney failure had progressed to the point that he could no longer work or drive, and his wife, Amanda, was considering suicide. While it was true that caring for Abe had become increasingly difficult, that was not Amanda's major problem. Much like Paul and Marilyn whom we met in chapter 3, the more Amanda did for her husband, the more he vituperated against her. "In his eyes, nothing I do is right," she complained. "I feel absolutely beaten down."

Abe and Amanda acted out their feelings, rather than expressing them in words. They usually didn't mean what they said to each other. My task was to act as interpreter: through me Abe and Amanda could express their feelings to each other. For example, when Abe criticized Amanda's driving, he really meant: "I'm unhappy and angry that I no longer have that privilege." When Amanda threatened to go away for a few days, she was really saying: "I need a brief respite and some support."

Even Amanda's suicide threats veiled her true needs; they were a cry for attention and appreciation from Abe for how hard she was working. Amanda never resented caring for her husband; she only resented never receiving thanks.

Once I began seeing them individually, it became clear how completely devoted Amanda was to Abe and how grateful he was for her care. I knew that Amanda would never put her husband in a nursing home to punish him for his behavior, although this was what he feared most. I also knew that in order to keep her happy, all that Abe need do was reward her kindness with a few words of appreciation.

However, a day didn't pass that Abe didn't test Amanda's loyalty. When he saw her frustration and exhaustion, he yelled at her, "Why don't you just put me in a nursing home?"—even though he was truly terrified that she would. He worried every time she went out (including if it was only to the grocery or church) that she wouldn't return or that she would be making plans for his institutionalization behind his back. Behind his constant snarls resided his irrational fear that she might one day abandon him.

My task was to show Abe and Amanda how to read between the lines—to see what was going on behind the obvious behavior. I had them ask themselves: "When he/she acts this way, what is he/she trying to tell me? What does he/she really mean?"

Not surprisingly, after several sessions, Abe and Amanda's relationship improved. Abe stopped disparaging his wife. He even organized their children to help her run the household without him. But his very best gesture was to buy her a small gold bracelet as a surprise on their anniversary. The bracelet was inexpensive—they couldn't afford much with Abe unable to work—but it was worth more than its weight in gold, for it was a constant reminder to Amanda, no matter how tough their situation, that Abe appreciated her devotion.

In turn, Amanda learned that Abe needed her verbal assurances that she still loved him and would never leave him, along with the good physical care she was giving him.

TAKING CHARGE OF YOUR
FEAR OF ABANDONMENT

Sharing adversity is one of the best things family members do for one another. This time, you may need your loved ones' help, but perhaps in the future, someone may need you—even simply to relieve his or her guilt. If you can accept this, then there are a number of ways you can help yourself deal with your fears.

- Keep in mind who is the culprit.
- Don't misinterpret family communications.
- Before conquering your fear, you must confront it.
- Discuss your fears with your loved ones.
- Be sensitive to your family's needs.
- Become aware of your own negative feelings.
- Express empathy and appreciation.
- Remain emotionally involved.
- Have realistic expectations.
- Remember, feelings are temporary.
- Be realistic about alternatives to home care.

Let's look at these steps in more detail.

Keep in Mind Who Is the Culprit

You and your family must recognize and accept that the disease—and not you—is at the root of the problem. Then your discussions and actions can be constructive. Remember, your family may wish to be free of the burden of the illness, not you.

Don't Misinterpret Family Communications

Family members may communicate that they need respite but you may believe they want a permanent escape.

If you fear that your spouse wishes to be "rid" of you because you are "demanding," you may be misreading the situation. He may be overwrought, even tired of your demands, but may need only a short respite or your expression of appreciation for his efforts. Becoming conscious of possible misinterpretations helps avoid this confusion and its negative consequences.

Before Conquering Your Fear, You Must Confront It

The fear of abandonment is normal, as is the difficulty in discussing it. Once you understand this, you can transfer the blame for the situation from your own shoulders to where it rightly belongs—the illness itself. Doing this immediately reduces your anxiety, making it easier for you to come up with your own solutions. For example, I never suggested any solutions to Joe and Amanda. I didn't have to. Once they confronted their fears and understood their feelings, they were able to devise their own innovative solutions to problems that arose in their family.

Discuss Your Fears with Your Loved Ones

It's important for you to explain to your family what you're frightened of and to ask for reassurance if you need it. Since your survival may depend on your ability to discuss this difficult issue, do not waver in your resolve to bring your feelings out into the open. At the same time, however, don't forget what your loved ones can tolerate. Even if your fears seem irrational, it's still better that you and your family face them down.

If you want to bring up your fears but find it difficult to do so openly, use whatever words feel comfortable at the moment. You could say, "Right now, I'm feeling lonely. Do you think you could go to the grocery store later?"

You may not be directly on target, but you won't be too far from the truth.

If you are at ease being completely open, you can make the simple admission "I'm really scared!" Explain what is frightening you. Your family will almost certainly understand your feelings because they are legitimate.

Some individuals are terrified to show their vulnerability. Just bear in mind that rather than lowering others' opinions of you, openness leads to mutual respect and empathy. Your family knows it's hard for you to share your worst fears. You need to recognize that it's equally hard for them to discuss theirs. Nevertheless, bringing up these apprehensions won't make them happen and may even alleviate them.

If all you need is reassurance, ask your family for it. But understand that constantly testing your family's limits can backfire. It may lead to hostility and may make your worst fear—abandonment—come true.

If your immediate family is frightened of hearing about your fears, you may push them to the point of rebellion. It's best under these circumstances to find someone else—a parent, sibling, counselor, or friend—to confide in. It's vital to understand others' limits.

Be Sensitive to Your Family's Needs

Your loved ones may be genuinely tired. You will benefit directly if you can sense when your family needs rest and can communicate your understanding to them. If nothing else, they'll be more willing to help you. If at all possible, urge them to take some time off. Besides, if you initiate the discussion, it will relieve your family of the guilt of having to bring it up.

Monitor your family's situation. Ask them, "Are you tired? Am I pushing too hard? Is this too much for you? If so, tell me what I can do and I'll try to be less demanding."

You may not get clear, honest statements because your loved ones may fear hurting your feelings. In that case, you could put words in their mouths. You might say, for example, "It has to be tiring for you to take care of me. It would be tiring for me! It's OK. I understand." In that way, you will help your loved ones feel that they are not trapped.

If you can, negotiate specific solutions to your situation. For example, let your caretaker go out with your permission, encouragement, and even insistence—without guilt. If possible, give your caregiver a day off once a week to go to the beauty parlor, play a round of golf, or have lunch with a friend. See if other family members, neighbors, or friends can take over the caretaker's responsibilities for a couple of hours. If your loved ones can share the caring, they will still feel valuable and needed, but some of the individual responsibility will be diminished.

Get out as much as possible on your own. This will help your family recognize your ability to care for yourself. If that's impossible, research resources in the community that might provide your family with a break. Here are a few suggestions:

- Seek out community activities or services provided by hospitals or social service agencies.
- Look for separate, "outside" activities—book review circles, movies, lectures, or concerts—that you might enjoy for several hours at a time without the need for your caregiver.
- Read newsletters published by community health agencies. These excellent resources can provide you with other activities.
- Informational films and discussion groups can also give you tips on how others have dealt with your dilemmas.

When you do the research, you save your family time while demonstrating to them that you want to help them get some relief. In addition, when you're engaged in these kinds of activities, you remain in charge as you relieve your family of some of the burden of your care.

Become Aware of Your Own Negative Feelings

What if, rather than encouraging your family to take some rest, you sabotage their efforts? For example, you may tell them that you want them to take time for themselves, but as they get ready to go, you blurt out "When will you be back? Will you be home at eight to give me my medicine?" or "I don't feel well. Do you really have to go tonight?"

Ask yourself why you are undermining your loved ones' time off. You might discover feelings you don't like in yourself, such as jealousy or resentment. These are not bad per se; they are normal. But you don't have to act on them. You simply have to recognize them. In the long run, this self-examination helps your family, but it helps you even more. If, to their delight, you offer loved ones respite and then renege, you are risking their deep disappointment—even anger.

Express Empathy and Appreciation

Your caregivers will feel more inclined to help out when they feel understood and valued. Whereas your criticism and anger may drive them away, your sincere expression of sympathy for their position will relieve all of you of pressures and misunderstandings. You might say, for instance, "I know how you feel. There are days when you're just fed up. I understand!" Your sensitivity will go a long way toward alleviating any hard feelings that may be building.

By the same token, it is advisable to allow family members to ventilate their frustrations with assurances of your understanding. Ask how you can help. If you determine that you need an outside party to mediate, seek one out. You might consider a therapist, member of the clergy, or other trusted and experienced individual to help you all sort through your complex feelings.

Remain Emotionally Involved

Maintain your role in the family. You are still a vital member, despite your illness. If you pull away, fearing you have become a burden or in preparation for an imagined or anticipated rejection, your loved ones may misinterpret your coolness and withdraw in response.

Have Realistic Expectations

Your family may have reached its limit and be giving all they can. Some people are better able to manage than others. For example, you may realize that in your marriage you have always been a caretaker. If so, that means your partner is unaccustomed to taking over and may be unable to manage the household or the finances.

If you are continually disappointed in your spouse's performance, you will become chronically frustrated, angry, and dissatisfied. He, in turn, will feel inadequate and unable to meet your demands. You may hear your spouse saying, for instance, "No matter what I do, it's never good enough!"

It's best to focus on what your caregiver *can* do, rather than on where he is deficient, and then to let go. Your implicit or explicit criticism can cause your loved one to eventually withdraw, the consequence you fear the most.

Remember, Feelings Are Temporary

Your caregiver may feel more tired and frustrated than you. She may feel that you are overdemanding and inconsiderate. She may even say "I don't know how much more of this I can take." You, on the other hand, may feel that you are responsive to her needs and do not ask too much.

Yet, although your caregiver may feel exhausted at one moment, some time later, she may be renewed. Emotions are temporary expressions of the moment. Indeed, when you look at feelings as transitory states, you need not be threatened by expressions of exhaustion or burdenedness. Use them as guides for you and your family—signals to let you all know that a situation needs to be altered. Here is where you'll all need to begin your changes.

Be Realistic About Alternatives to Home Care

Being moved into a nursing home may not constitute an abandonment but rather an act of caring and concern for your safety. If your family must consider alternatives to home care, become part of the discussion and decision early on.

Some individuals have their families *promise* that they will never send them to nursing homes. It's normal to ask for such reassurance and your family can feel good about making such a sincere pledge. However, in truth, no one knows what the future will bring. It may come to the point, after all alternatives have been exhausted, that there is no choice but institutionalization. In this case, bear in mind that placement is not necessarily abandonment. Release your family from the earlier promise and help them work through the guilt. As you have seen, although this is a difficult issue for many families, the ties of love and caring can be maintained even if physical problems must be treated outside the home. Love knows no walls.

REMEMBER

- The fear of being abandoned is universal and normal.
- When you're chronically ill, this fear intensifies.
- You may try to test your family's limits to see if they'll "stay," but this can be damaging.
- It can be difficult and confusing to share your fears with your loved ones.
- Sometimes we believe or fear that we are being abandoned, when in reality, we are not.
- Your family may want to be rid of your disease—not you.
- Feelings are temporary.

THINGS TO DO

- Be careful not to misinterpret family communications.
- Confront your fear before trying to conquer it.
- Discuss your fears with your loved ones.
- Be sensitive to your family's needs.
- Become aware of your own negative feelings.
- Express empathy and appreciation.
- Remain emotionally involved.
- Have realistic expectations, especially about home care.

10.

Mastering Your Fear of Expressing Anger

Anger is often difficult to recognize and acknowledge in oneself. You pay dearly when you cover your anger, trying to appear cool and controlled when you're not.

I know this from personal experience. I had no idea how much anger had affected my life—I didn't even know that I was angry. Some of my friends recognized it in me, but when one of my confidants mentioned that she thought I must be pretty enraged at what had happened to my family, I reacted as if she were crazy. "How dare she think I'm angry," I thought. "I'm upset and unhappy because of my children's deaths, but angry? Never."

Of course, I sometimes felt that my life was over—I had put so much of it into my futile attempts at saving my sick youngsters. And certainly, I had asked myself repeatedly why two innocent children had to be born with such serious illnesses and had to suffer so. I wondered why all of my friends seemed to be able to give birth to one healthy baby after another, while two of my three biological children were so terribly sick. I questioned if there was anything I had done to cause my children's pain, for I was certain that they had no responsibility in it. These concerns plagued me for years, yet I never recognized that I was angry about them.

Indeed, I realized that sometimes I was impatient and short with my family. Even though I didn't like showing my emotions—I felt embarrassed by them and their intensity—they spilled over. When I tried to contain them, I became depressed and developed a series of psychosomatic complaints such as dizziness and severe backaches that were not properly diagnosed at that time.

In addition, I felt deeply disappointed in close family and friends who seemed to misunderstand me. I used to ask myself, "Don't they know how terrible I feel? Can't they read me?" On many occasions, I sat in one room feeling as if my world had fallen apart, while my husband and surviving children laughed at a TV sitcom or cheered a sporting event in an adjoining room. If, in my state of upset, I came out to talk to them about my feelings, they gave me strange looks rather than sympathy or support. I needed their love and understanding, but felt, instead, isolated, insecure, and "crazy."

Sometimes the frustration became so intense that I became desperate. At times, I believed I could no longer handle life. I could see no way to better my situation; whatever I did seemed wrong. As my family lost respect for me, I lost respect for myself. They began treating my outbursts as wild ravings; I had increasingly lost control over my life.

My family, like those of so many of my patients these days, must have felt that I had changed. I knew I hadn't. Inside, I was still the same person, but I was hurting so much that I had no way to express it.

Moreover, my attempts at hiding my rage and pain made outsiders believe that I was cold and detached. Because they never saw me crying, they thought I always had my life together. But that wasn't my reality. In truth, I appeared calm because I was on tranquilizers for nine years. During this period, I did have some bursts of erratic behavior, but most of the time, I actually felt very little. My doctors' idea, of course, was to get me through this difficult period, but in fact (as I realized later) the medication delayed my undergoing a process that was vital to my recovery.

Without working through my anger, I could never resolve my grief. Once I faced these feelings, I could regain control of my life. Yet, with the tranquilizers, the anger just sat in my guts, increasing in intensity as the years went by. Like one of my patients said of herself, "I had a scream just waiting to get out." My problem back then was that I didn't know how to release it safely.

ANGER IS A NORMAL BUT MISUNDERSTOOD EMOTION

Anger is so often misunderstood. As you can see from my experience, when left untended, it has the potential for becoming destructive; expressed inappropriately, it can be equally so.

Some people think of anger as bad or a dirty word. They hide their feelings because expressing them in the past had caused them guilt or had undermined important relationships. Perhaps their parents had always lectured them to be nice and get along, even if they felt wronged by friends or siblings. Others, rather than hiding their anger, may explode with rage, unable to manage its intensity. Some men fear anger, because it may indicate that they are out of control. Some women are afraid to express it because they don't want to appear unfeminine. Many individuals deny it, as I did.

Anger is a normal response to frustration. And who doesn't deal with some form of frustration every single day of his or her life? Who doesn't wish to get through rush-hour traffic faster or talk to the person he or she phoned, instead of voice mail? The very idea of a long-term illness—something you can do very little about—is the epitome of frustration. *If anger is a response to frustration, you can see how it is natural to feel angry when you must cope with a chronic disease.*

The list of frustrations is long and unending, the major one being the illness's unpredictable and incurable nature. This is particularly difficult in our society, where we believe that somewhere, somehow, there surely is a remedy for what ails us, and furthermore, that it was in our power to prevent disease in the first place.

One of my patients stated this frustration most succinctly when she said, "I don't understand! I did all the right things. How could I get sick?" Perhaps this attitude is rooted in the belief that if we eat the right foods, get enough exercise, stop smoking, and reduce stress we can live "forever"—well, maybe not forever, but certainly to a ripe old age! Unfortunately, as you well know, that is not always the case.

HOW LONG-TERM ILLNESS MAKES YOU ANGRY

There is no question that you will feel angry if you have taken good care of your body all your life and you *still* become ill. If you actively work to avoid illness, only to discover that you were powerless to stop it, you experience the ultimate frustration.

On the other hand, if you feel that you could have done better, that somehow you slipped up, you may believe that you have caused your disease. When you take the blame, you become angry with yourself. Or you may believe that you have been a good person all your life, but made one transgression, and now you're being punished for it. Why else would this terrible thing happen? In this case, you might feel like a victim.

"Why me?" you may be wondering. "Why now? . . .

- ". . . Just when I was getting ready to retire and finally do the traveling I've been waiting for."
- ". . . Just when I got married and landed a great job."
- ". . . Just when I wanted to have lots of kids."

"What did I do to deserve this?" You believe that you have been dealt a bad hand, and you feel sorry for yourself.

THE DYNAMICS OF FREE-FLOATING ANGER

OK, so anger is a given in your situation. How do you deal with it? Some people turn their rage outward, at everyone around them. Anyone who looks at them funny gets zapped. Barbara described, for example, how, when her husband walked in the house after a long day at work, instead of throwing her arms around him and kissing him, she yelled at him for forgetting to buy the milk for tomorrow's breakfast. She risked alienating the one person who cared for her the most. Such indiscriminate expression of anger may garner temporary relief, but in the long run, it can only exacerbate an already tense situation.

Others may turn their rage inward, against themselves, and become severely depressed. Rita was sitting in a restaurant enjoying an intimate evening with her good friends, when suddenly, and "inexplicably," she felt tears rolling down her cheeks. She couldn't stop them. By directing her anger at herself, she risked depression (to the point of considering suicide) and a stress-induced increase of her physical symptoms.

Besides, if you remain silent or are simply seething inside without letting your feelings out, you will frustrate those around you. They will sense that you're angry, but they won't know why, or if they had anything to do with it.

As you can see, none of these strategies are helpful. As often happens with long-term illnesses, both Barbara and Rita were dealing with anger that had been misplaced; it was directed at the wrong target. *Even though they couldn't verbalize their true feelings, deep down inside, they were both angry at their illnesses.* Because most people don't realize that the real origin of their rage is their disease, they focus it on other sources: doctors, family, friends, children, themselves. After all, they can't yell at their damaged heart muscle, lungs, or kidneys.

This *free-floating* anger needs a focus to help relieve the inner tension it creates. Your asthma may not react to you, but if you yell at your wife, she will respond. You may experience some relief, but your wife's reaction may serve to heighten your tension and stress further.

TAKING CHARGE OF YOUR ANGER

Anger is a symptom of the way you feel, not the cause. Like all emotions, it is temporary. Your task is to find a way to express it that helps rather than hurts you. You already have learned that you can control your behavior. Similarly, how you cope with your anger is also in your hands. Taking charge will require that you discriminate how you ventilate these powerful feelings without upsetting everyone around you. But once you know how to express your anger appropriately, it will work to your advantage, not your detriment. Once you direct your rage at its true source—your illness— you can use it to serve you.

The benefits of doing so are many. When you come to terms with your anger, you will begin to feel hopeful; you'll increase your energy, maintain family relations, and find peace of mind. You might even slow the progress of your illness.

In order to master your fear of anger, you'll need to take the following steps:

- Begin with self-evaluation.
- Assess your feelings about anger.
- Expect your anger to surface.
- Note where you are focusing your rage.
- Give yourself and everyone else a break.
- Use words to express your feelings.
- Find a safe place to vent your emotions.
- Be creative in finding outlets for your anger.
- Take into account your family's anger.
- Accept your situation.

Let's look at these steps in more detail.

Begin with Self-evaluation

The first step in overcoming your fear of anger is to recognize rage in yourself. That's not always as easy as it sounds.

"Well," you might say, "I'm *really* not angry. It's true that sometimes I'm upset, short-tempered, or lethargic. And sometimes I feel completely hopeless, even to the point of considering suicide. Yes, there are moments when I feel no one cares about me and that there's no light at the end of the tunnel. I do wonder why I, of all people, have been singled out for this terrible fate, but I'm not angry. I may be depressed."

In truth, these feelings are easier to admit than rage, yet they mask the anger beneath them. It helps to recognize them as such. Remember, depression is simply anger turned inward.

To evaluate if you are experiencing anger, ask yourself: How do you express your anger? Do you hold it in or blow it out? Do you gnash your teeth or scream or seethe inwardly? Can you recognize when you're feeling depressed (some of the symptoms include feeling tired, listless, "bad," anguished, unmotivated, or lacking in appetite)? Or do you feel as if you're in a prison cell with the walls closing in? Do you feel that it would it be easier to give up than go on? If you are depressed, you can be sure you are suppressing your anger.

Assess Your Feelings About Anger

Many of my patients have denied or feared their anger. In order to take charge, it will help to analyze what preconceptions you may have toward this emotion.

How was anger treated in your family when you were growing up? Could you express your feelings easily in words such as "I'm furious!" or did you have to hide your true emotions? Did your parents scold you with statements such as "You don't act that way in this family!" Indeed, how acceptable was it for you to express your feelings as a child? Was it a family value to avoid talking about "these things"? Is it easier to admit to depression? Is it terrible to be angry? Answers to these questions may give you a clue as to why you sometimes feel that you are bursting or why you feel it would be awful to just "let it all out."

Expect Your Anger to Surface

You can count on your anger surfacing. It will make itself known directly or indirectly. If suppressed, it will build in intensity until it erupts. In fact, the longer you wait to express it, the larger the explosion becomes. Contained, anger has the potential for causing the kind of psychological and psychosomatic symptoms I myself experienced.

If you accept anger as a natural consequence of long-term illness, you can release it constructively and with a measure of control.

A note here on tranquilizers: Unwittingly, many doctors buy into their patients' fear of anger by prescribing these medications to mask the feelings. Be wary of this. Drugs may calm you for the moment, but they will not alleviate the deeper problem. They may simply delay the natural process that you must experience in order to take charge of your life.

Note Where You Are Focusing Your Rage

Free-floating anger may alight on anyone nearby—family, friends, doctors. Are you using a person or an institution as an object of your intense feelings? Is it some family member whom you feel doesn't understand your changed behavior? Your boss? Your son's teacher? Your daughter-in-law?

Ask yourself: Who or what am I angry at, *really?*

Give Yourself and Everyone Else a Break

Don't allow yourself to be angry with yourself. I call this the "double whammy." In addition to coping with your disease, you're adding an extra burden by believing that you are part of the problem. In order to get on with your life, you must take responsibility for the future without blaming yourself for the past.

To the best of your ability, remove the blame for your illness from yourself or some other source, and place it squarely where it belongs—on the environment or genetics. Be realistic. How much control did you really have over what happened? Could you have prevented it in any way? Perhaps hindsight is tormenting you. Tell yourself what you want to hear: that you did the best you could at the moment.

Be reassured that even if your anger appears ugly sometimes, loved ones can understand it, especially if you explain why it occurred or if you can prepare them in advance by saying "Right now, I'm so angry, I feel like hitting, screaming, or cursing!"

Don't expect others to understand your behavior without some explanation from you. Unless they have personally experienced your situation, they really don't have the same frame of reference. Explain your actions and emotions to your loved ones so they will understand your predicament.

Use Words to Express Your Feelings

Anger can be understood, tolerated, and discussed. For example, begin by explaining why it's so important for you to express your anger. Ask for indulgence and help. Tell your family that it feels awkward for you to be angry, but you know that you must. You can even explain that you're not exactly sure why you feel this way, but you'd like their forebearance as you go through this difficult process.

You can also explain to your loved ones that all you want is an ear. You don't need them to solve your problems—they may be unable to, anyway. But their listening will give you a chance to release some of your pent-up feelings. It's something positive they can do for you.

In your discussion, simple expressions like "I feel so frustrated!" or "Sometimes I feel sorry for myself!" or "I'm just enraged!" help to break the ice without explosive outbursts that can be dangerous to you. You are describing how you feel without blaming anyone. And your loved ones will respond, but without an argument. They won't feel attacked or need to defend themselves. After you have expressed your anger, its intensity will have diminished and you will regain a sense of control.

Be careful when you speak that you don't say things that can never be retracted or forgiven. Find a way to express yourself that's judicious and safe for you. When you explain yourself to loved ones, use "I" statements about your feelings (such as "I feel hurt when you don't call") rather than "you" statements (such as "How dare you not call!"). Your friends and family will experience the latter as a form of verbal aggression and will become defensive. Anger dumped indiscriminately may bring temporary relief but can permanently damage relationships you really care about. "I" statements will garner a more positive response (see pp. 48–52 for other helpful communication skills).

Finally, observe if your words and actions are in sync with your feelings. If you watch yourself, you may discover that you are one of those individuals (like me) who hide their true feelings. I learned that people often misread me because I continued to smile, even when I spoke of painful subjects. How could others know that I was hurting when my demeanor gave them a different message? While you may think that you are expressing how you feel, you may be conveying mixed messages. Make sure that those with whom you communicate fully understand you.

Find a Safe Place to Vent Your Emotions

If your family cannot tolerate a discussion of feelings, especially anger, but you need that release, then you might make use of a peer support group offered through community health agencies. You will be welcomed with open arms, and you will no longer feel alone or embarrassed by your emotions. At a support group, you will learn that the world hasn't turned against you.

The support you receive will help you deal with your family. They may very well be experiencing their own anger, and acting it out against you. They too may feel helpless, alone, and/or frustrated. They may be irritated at being forced into a role they cannot or don't want to handle. Listen to their complaints (which are probably much the same as yours). Help them to release their frustrations. Family support groups can be a safe place for your loved ones to let go of some of their pent-up feelings.

Be Creative in Finding Outlets for Your Anger

You might try some of these suggestions to manage your anger:

1. If you feel you're going to blow up, give yourself a time-out. Use the old-fashioned "count to ten." Walk out of the room if you must. This gives you time and space to think things through. One wise couple handled this situation extremely well. When their situation became tense, Eleanor left the house since Warren was in a wheelchair. She visited a friend, went to a movie, or took a long drive. They both knew what they were doing and why.

Marge had a different solution. She used her car as a private space. She turned the radio volume up full blast and screamed as loud as she could. When she felt better, she returned home to her waiting family.

Find your own way. Punch a pillow. Jump up and down. Yell at a houseplant. Talk back to the TV. Release the tension in a way that feels safe for you.

2. Give yourself sympathy if no one else will. I believe in a little self-pity, a little wallowing around, a little feeling sorry for yourself. When you believe no one cares about your situation, treat yourself well; give yourself a little sympathy. But notice that I said "a little." You need to know when to stop. If you've been lying around in bed all day, get up. Take a shower, spray perfume. Pamper yourself. Soothe and nourish yourself.

3. Forgive and understand the insensitivity or clumsiness of others. It's likely that many people will respond to you insensitively: they will say the wrong things and hurt your feelings. Rather than harboring anger against them (which does you little good), forgive and understand their ignorance and clumsiness. They have probably never experienced anything like your trauma.

I remember feeling incensed at people who were patronizing and tactless. I would think, "What do they know of my pain?" I was right; they didn't know about it. But it would have been better for me if I understood that I had been displacing my anger about my daughter's death onto these individuals. They didn't deserve all the rage I was dishing out to them. They were limited, as we all are, and were doing the best that they could to console me.

4. Take action. Once you have redirected your energy away from suppressing your anger, you'll find that you can use your newfound vitality to your benefit. Ask more questions about your illness. Do your own research. Learn more about your prognosis and the latest treatments available. In this way, you will take more control of medical decisions you must make.

As you do this, recognize that you are releasing your anger constructively. Even if you get a worst-case scenario from your physician as you probe further and further—one that might never occur—this still allows you to plan your life more effectively. You will no longer fear the unknown and can then take charge of your life.

5. *Make lists.* As I suggested in chapter 6, you can list your losses. This will help you to see exactly how many and what they are. Then you can focus even more on what you're really angry about. You might evaluate each loss as to whether it's permanent or transitory, and if there is anything you can do about it.

Why not list ways to use energy positively once your depression lifts? Itemize workable and unworkable ideas, the ideal and the real. But take action only on the realistic ones, so you can see some results. You might think of raising money for research, influencing public policy, or organizing people and services to help others who are similarly afflicted. These activities will help others in your position who don't have your wisdom or understanding.

Take Into Account Your Family's Anger

It is quite likely that your family will experience anger about the situation you all find yourselves in. To help you cope with their emotions, you might ask yourself the following questions:

- Is my family angry too?
- Do they keep their feelings inside?
- Do they direct their rage at me (rather than the disease)?
- How does my spouse express his anger?
- Where can he go with it if he feels he can't let it out with me?
- Can we share our common anger and grow from it?

Just as you need to vent your rage safely, it's important for your loved ones to have permission and a time and place for their emotions. They can benefit from the suggestions I've given you, and may also derive solace from family peer support groups.

Accept Your Situation

Your anger can work for or against you. It's up to you to decide which it will be. You have the power to control your behavior. No matter how much you may feel a victim, you need not be.

The key for me was embracing my anger. Once I realized that I no longer feared being angry or expressing this emotion, I freed myself from its hold. I began to accept my destiny—the events in my life that I was powerless to change. Genetics and nature had determined my children's health. As much as I would have wished that circumstances be otherwise, I had little to do with it. As my elderly aunt Bertha used to say, "Man plans and God laughs."

Once I came to this feeling of acceptance, I again took charge of my life. I began making decisions about what I wanted to do with the rest of my time. I returned to school, got a master's degree in social work, worked as a therapist, and wrote this book. In the process, I discovered energy that I believed I had lost forever.

I no longer felt alone in my suffering. I particularly remember two questions that I had asked myself toward the end of this process. The first: "Do you think you're the only one in the world with these problems?" I knew that they were unusual, but I also knew that others must have struggled with them too. Then I asked myself: "Did you think you could go through life unscathed by illness and tragedy?" I answered, "I had hoped so. Who doesn't?" But I also knew that I was part of the human race. Whatever the rest of humanity was prone to, I might also experience.

Once I had reached this point, I realized that I had accepted what was given and was no longer angry about it. My self-pitying lament, "Why me?" became a more realistic "Why not me?"

ELLEN VENTS HER ANGER

Ellen, a woman in her early forties, had hidden her anger for so many years that, when she was forced to deal with cancer, her rage almost did her in. She did not understand her intense feelings, nor did she accept them.

Prior to her diagnosis of breast cancer, Ellen had stock-piled anger from her adolescence. Mostly focused on her parents, it had remained hidden and unresolved for almost thirty years. With the advent of cancer, however, it intensified and spread. Now, Ellen directed her rage at her husband and young son. She had always concealed her rage from her parents and friends (they knew her as quiet and shy), but now it was spilling over. At home, she was out of control.

Not that Ellen didn't have plenty to be angry about. At thirty-six she had been diagnosed with cervical cancer; she immediately had a hysterectomy. Now, four years later, she had gotten breast cancer. Going through a second round of chemotherapy, she again was losing her hair and feeling sick from the treatments.

Like so many others, Ellen did not ascertain the source of her feelings. She turned her anger first on herself, and then on her loved ones. During our first meeting, she announced, "I caused my cancer! I have a terrible personality! If I had been a different person, my life might have turned out better!" What a terrible burden to lay on one's back. Ellen felt unlovable. Indeed, if people did give her compliments, she believed they didn't really mean it.

Her home, the very place where she needed to seek solace for her woes, became a battleground. She didn't blame her husband and son for her illness, but they became the targets of her misdirected anger. They felt the full brunt of it until they could stand it no longer. After constant exposure to her invective, Ellen's family coped by avoiding her. They simply withdrew.

Ellen's pain was obvious. She loved her family but couldn't seem to control her destructive behavior. She might spend weeks trying to please them, but then in one night of rage she could destroy all of the good feelings she had worked so hard to develop. She was desperate.

How was I to help her? First, I believed that, before she could manage it, Ellen needed to see more clearly what had caused her incredible anger. We needed to relieve some of the stress in her life.

We began with Ellen's childhood. She still had mixed feelings about her parents. She loved them and felt that they had always been good to her, but she disapproved of their life-style. She found them too materialistic and ostentatious. She thought of herself as more intellectual and preferred remaining in the background. She had never resolved these differences with her parents, even though she accepted them for who they were (and by the same token, herself for who she was).

In our work together, Ellen realized that even though there were major philosophical differences, she adored her folks. In truth, they were very good to her and admired her. Telephone calls with her parents, formerly extremely tense, were now warm and friendly.

This issue resolved, we went on to others. Another stressful area in Ellen's life was her work. Although her job as an account executive in an advertising agency was pressure filled, the work itself did not cause her great stress. Rather, she felt unable to deal with some of her colleagues.

It was not easy, but Ellen agreed to make some changes in order to alleviate her tension.

She quit her job and took a much needed and long delayed vacation. Then she found a new position at a different advertising agency. She even tried some relaxation techniques, such as yoga, biofeedback, and meditation. I admired her for attempting these, because they felt alien to her. After a while, she began to see their value.

We had an excellent relationship, and Ellen was making some strides in understanding and controlling her anger. She had even reduced some of her stress. But then, one day, seemingly out of the blue, a rage that I had only heard about turned directly toward me.

"You're not doing enough for me," Ellen railed. "I want to see some other therapists." From the way she spoke, it was clear that she was denigrating me personally. In her eyes, I wasn't good enough.

I was surprised, but I let Ellen continue her thirty-minute tirade. As her face began turning red and the pitch of her voice sharpened, I realized that she was awaiting my response. As calmly as I could, I said, "It is your prerogative to change therapists, but it is not necessary for you to insult or disparage me. You are angry. I understand. But I am not the source of your frustration. Your illness is. You can leave now, if you want to."

When Ellen walked out the door, I was sure I would never see her again. However, the following week, at her appointed hour, there she was in my waiting room (I hadn't yet filled her time slot with another patient). Again, I was surprised, but once in my office, Ellen was her old self. She apologized with as much charm and warmth as I knew her capable of.

In trying to understand why the outburst had occurred, I realized that the stress-reducing strategies we had followed had helped Ellen with her life but did little for her disease.

I could do nothing in that area for her. In her frustration, she vented her anger about her illness on me. And so, we finally got down to the source of Ellen's rage. She took the first step, by admitting her anger. It put the issue within her control.

I said, "You know, I am only able to help you in certain ways. I wish I could help in others. But now that you know why you're so angry, you can do what you want with your feelings. You can release it on your family, like you had, or on a bank clerk, if you feel like it. Or you can express it in words, and let it out safely. It's up to you."

Ellen understood, and we continued our work. She improved. Even though she still did occasionally feel the frustration of being powerless about her illness, she managed to do a lot about her life and the relationships that meant the most to her. The explosions directed at her husband and son diminished, and for the first time in her life, she felt loved and lovable. She was directing her anger at its true source.

In fact, just before she completed treatment, Ellen gave herself a gift: a Valentine's party. It was a last-minute idea, but she pulled it off with aplomb. All her friends came to help her celebrate her new lease on life. The party was Ellen's way of marking the changes in insight and behavior: from all-consuming work to time for pleasure; from a choking anger that almost destroyed all that she had loved to a sense of mastery and control. Ellen's party was a sign to her that she was no longer her anger's victim.

You too can learn lessons from Ellen's experience. When your anger is focused on its real source, you gain the advantage of being in charge of your life. Your illness might have altered your life, but you are still in control of how you run it. Anger represents energy that, once released, can serve you. After you have subdued your rage, you will find yourself making clearer decisions that are vital to your survival.

REMEMBER

- Anger is often difficult to recognize and acknowledge in yourself.
- You pay dearly when you cover your anger and try to appear cool and controlled when you're not.
- Anger is a normal emotion and an expectable consequence of chronic illness.
- Free-floating anger can be misdirected at friends and loved ones or at yourself.
- Depression is anger turned inward.
- Tranquilizers can mask real emotions and delay their resolution.

THINGS TO DO

- Evaluate yourself.
- Assess your feelings about anger.
- Expect anger to surface.
- Note where you are focusing your rage.
- Give yourself and everyone else a break.
- Use words to express your feelings.
- Find a place to vent your emotions.
- Be creative in finding outlets for your anger.
- Accept your situation.

11.

Mastering Your Fear of Isolation

Sandra, a young blind woman, explained to me how isolating her condition was for her. One day, she and a group of sighted friends went out for lunch. Within a few minutes of being seated, the waiter came over and took everyone's order but hers. Finally, after an awkward pause, he asked no one in particular, "And, what does *she* want to eat?"

Sandra knew the waiter was talking about her, and she was angry that he hadn't spoken directly to her. She remained silent in face of the slight, but to me she said, "Just because I can't see, it doesn't mean I can't think or talk! I was so embarrassed. I felt denigrated, as if I were less of a person. Situations like these make me want to stay home and never go out with my sighted friends. How else can I avoid getting hurt and humiliated like this?"

I explained to her that I was sure the waiter knew she could think and talk. My guess was that he was anxious about getting her attention. Perhaps he felt uncomfortable reaching over the person closest to him in the booth to tap Sandra on the shoulder. ("Besides," I asked, "wouldn't you have been even more embarrassed had he singled you out in that way?") Worried about how to handle this potentially unpleasant situation, the waiter seemed to choose the easiest route for him—he referred to Sandra in the third person. Despite his best intentions, however, his actions had a negative effect on this young woman. They seemed to reinforce her feelings of isolation.

I have found that people coping with long-term illnesses often retreat into their homes or some other safe, supportive environment, much as Sandra was tempted to do. Understandably, they choose to be with people with whom they feel comfortable: those who are nonthreatening and to whom they need not explain their condition or their feelings. Once in the cocoon, they receive empathy and understanding. What could be better?

Unfortunately, there is a down side to this withdrawal. Often, before they even realize what has happened, these people discover they have completely isolated themselves from the outside world. They have lost contact with old friends; they no longer participate in favorite activities or work. Their whole world shrinks, revolving exclusively around their illness and their inner circle of family and allies.

Why would anyone retreat in this way? It's actually easy. It feels better and safer to be with people who share your problem. Underlying this need for safety is a more painful truth: the fear of rejection. Of course, everyone, healthy or sick, fears rejection—it's a normal human emotion. However, this fear intensifies with one's diagnosis because of the possibility of being stigmatized (see chapter 8). The fear of rejection can be based on painful experiences that you've had or have witnessed. For many, it just seems easier to go into seclusion.

HOW ISOLATION BUILDS

There are actually several different kinds of isolation resulting from long-term illness: physical, social, and emotional. These build one upon the other.

For some ailments, *physical isolation* is almost a given. Some individuals are confined to their beds or their homes. Others must rely on wheelchairs or walkers to get around. Even though so many public places now accommodate them, these large mechanical devices are still encumbering. They make getting out and about difficult, especially since they often require that one be accompanied.

Such physical obstacles may curtail your outings, so you may have fewer social contacts. This can lead to *social isolation*, which is much more subtle than physical isolation, and therefore more difficult to overcome.

Immediately after your diagnosis, you may be deluged with phone calls, get-well notes, and flowers. These you welcome, but after a time you notice that the attention dwindles. Old friends may avoid you because of their discomfort at being unable to offer solutions or reassurance. They may feel sad and helpless about changes they see in you. Since they are uncomfortable, they may find it easier to stay away or stop calling.

Believing that your friends no longer care about you, you may see fewer and fewer of them, and increasingly withdraw into yourself. You may begin to fear others' insensitivity, their questioning looks, their excluding or ignoring you in conversation or decision making.

In truth, it is difficult to watch people pull away, especially those who are the closest. If you continue to dodge the inevitable confrontation of social rejection, a slow and insidious shift occurs. From others avoiding you, you may find that you begin to avoid others. *Emotional isolation*, perhaps your worst fear, has set in.

Emotional isolation causes the most anxiety and the deepest pain. When you're hurt, it's natural to withdraw, to give yourself time and space to lick your wounds before moving out into the world again. But you know that you have a more serious problem when you no longer wish to reach out; when you choose a safe but sequestered environment. When you become emotionally isolated, you may be forever estranged from familiar personal habits, friendships developed over a lifetime, and activities that have always meant a lot to you.

FAMILY MAY BECOME ISOLATED TOO

Your family members may also feel separated from others, reinforcing your state. Their self-confidence may be sorely tried at this time. They too may feel different and alienated from their friends. They may receive fewer phone calls and visits. They become aware that old friends have little understanding of their current problems and that they in turn have less and less in common with these friends.

Rachel, the mother of a seventeen-year-old paraplegic, described her disappointment in her friends after her son's tragic accident. "You know," she confided to me, "they have absolutely no idea of the personal pain I have been experiencing. I have found that I really prefer spending time with others who have suffered similar experiences to mine." As a consequence, Rachel withdrew from her pre-accident life.

PREPARING YOURSELF

Although you may resent having to take the responsibility, you are the best one to help yourself deal with isolation.

Better than anyone else, you understand why others may ignore or reject you. To avoid isolation, you must be ready to face the difficulties that may lie ahead.

In the event you believe someone is snubbing you, it may help for you to prepare a statement in advance. In dealing with Sandra's problem, for example, I asked her to think of ways she could handle flustered waiters. She decided she should project her voice and say "Maybe you missed me, but I want to order a burger and fries."

If she were able to deliver this statement with a smile, she would deal with the world without isolating herself from it. Still, it was most important for Sandra to be at ease with however she chose to react. If it felt better for her to allow the slight to pass uncommented upon, then she could await a future incident, when she was feeling more secure, to use her statement. Should she choose to remain silent, however, she still needed to anticipate that she might again feel rejected, hurt, angry, and embarrassed, although perhaps with less intensity.

Hanna's parents helped prepare her for the potential isolation that her condition might elicit. Born deaf, this young woman had spent much of her time in the world of the hearing impaired. However, her parents had insisted that she learn to speak. If she could only lip-read and use sign language, they reasoned, she would always be isolated. Speaking skills, although extremely difficult to acquire, would allow Hanna to perform ordinary activities, such as shopping in the supermarket, more easily. Hanna was quite clear when she told me, "I can't expect a grocery checker to know sign language."

Still, much like Sandra, Hanna was often subject to people ignoring or passing her by. In a group, individuals frequently spoke to one another, looking past her and making it impossible for her to lip-read. If she spoke, they often asked her to repeat herself. Sometimes, they even wanted to know if she had come from a foreign country. Because she had prepared herself for such slights, Hanna understood that these individuals didn't mean to hurt her feelings. They just didn't know what they needed to do to help her feel a part of the group. It was not personal rejection but ignorance.

Fortunately, Hanna had excellent support from her family, so she was able to roll with the punches. She saw that she had options. She could tell people how to include her or, if she felt the time and place weren't right, let the situation go. For example, she could say "I'm deaf. I'd appreciate it if you could speak more directly at me part of the time," or "I'm deaf. I hope you don't mind if I ask you to repeat some words. I don't want to miss anything you say."

"Sometimes," Hanna revealed, "I feel that I live in limbo, between the hearing impaired and the 'normal.' " But that didn't seem to stop her. She knew that she would always have to deal with some anxiety and rejection, but that was her choice. She decided that she could tolerate these feelings better than being isolated in the deaf world. She later married a man whose hearing was absolutely perfect.

THE PLEASURES
OF PEER SUPPORT GROUPS

You and your family need support. No one can cope with a chronic illness alone. In fact, isolation can only add to your problems. Community-based chapters of national organizations such as the American Cancer Society, the American Heart Association, the National Multiple Sclerosis Society, or the Wellness Community offer social opportunities, particularly peer support groups, as do hospital stroke and organ transplant clubs. They are open to everyone—patients and families—for free or for a very small fee. I am very familiar with these groups because over the years I have led them and recommended them to many of my patients.

Throughout this book, I have suggested peer support groups as a way to help you deal with your fears. When it comes to the issue of isolation, this advice can hold doubly true. The groups are often comfortable and comforting. Although most people approach them with some trepidation, usually they discover that they can feel safe and "among friends" there.

Group participants find that they need not explain themselves to others, since everyone else has had similar experiences. Feelings of differentness and alienation evaporate. In fact, sometimes, participants don't even need to speak if they're not up to it—sooner or later, someone else will voice their own concerns and thoughts. The people in the groups are supportive, and the atmosphere is inviting.

Support groups have many benefits:

1. Seeing survivors of the illness gives you hope. You may find, for example, that others in the group have had their illnesses longer than you have and they're coping well. They have survived and look better than you had any reason to expect they would. Their condition gives you hope that your disease will progress like theirs. Many a patient has reported back to me, "I couldn't tell the patients from the leaders."

On the other hand, sometimes as you listen to the coping strategies of others, you realize that you could never cope in their way. You would not want to. You like your own approach a whole lot better. This is also reinforcing and validating for you.

2. Sharing practical, emotional, and physical problems helps break the cycle of unwanted aloneness. New group members often gain valuable tips about how to manage their illness, their medical care, and their emotional lives. They learn from others who have already been through it about new treatments that may be available, and how to alleviate some of the discomforts they may be suffering. They learn how to deal with family and friends who may not understand their emotions.

3. Being able to laugh at mutual foibles and share painful experiences becomes healing. People who are tense and anxious about their illness-induced vulnerabilities in other settings may become comfortable and even jocular about them in a support group. For example, in a cancer group, those upset about having to wear wigs or scarves to cover their bare heads may pull them off with glee. Others laugh at shared experiences. Participants tell stories that are wonderfully funny in hindsight of incidents that were deeply embarrassing at the time—moments when they fell into someone's lap and were considered drunk, or when they wet their clothes waiting in a theater line because they couldn't get to a toilet.

A support group is one place in which you can roar with laughter at your problems. When you are feeling alone, different, rejected, or isolated, sharing painful experiences in this way can have an extraordinarily healing effect. It may even prolong your life.

4. It's safe. The atmosphere in peer support groups is one of complete security. It's the one place you'll never have to worry about being rejected. Often the kind of empathic support you'll receive can come only from outsiders, since your family members may be feeling as isolated and different as you are. Besides, members feel a genuine delight in your becoming part of the group. Many people who had feared their first session have walked out of it feeling warm, happy, and almost euphoric.

A Caveat

A peer support group can fill a deep void, especially if you have little family support available or if loved ones live far away. Groups can be a beacon of light, getting you through what may seem like your darkest hour.

However, although support groups sound like the best of all possible solutions, they should not in and of themselves become a permanent way of life for you. Becoming a participant in such a group does not replace your need for acceptance in the larger society. These groups offer wonderfully positive experiences when you're feeling needy and vulnerable, but at some point you must consider leaving this haven and rejoining your old friends and life.

Your goal should be clear when you enter a group: You want to return to as normal a way of life as possible, as soon as you can. You must integrate lessons learned and move on.

In order to do so, you'll need to decide how much support you need, and for how long. You may want to assess the group's value to you. Everyone differs in this regard, according to personality and family situations. Resources vary. Some individuals prefer getting support from friends, even if their family is quite available. Others need outside help for only a short time while still others require it for several years and even the rest of their lives. Any way you decide to get support is fine, as long as you recognize why you've made the decisions you have.

In extreme and rare cases, you may find that you feel like a traitor if you wish to leave the group. Members may subtly emphasize feelings of group cohesiveness and alienation in such statements as "The rest of the world is cruel and uncaring" or "Yeah, they just don't understand us." Vulnerable individuals may identify so strongly with the group that they further estrange themselves from the world at large. As one of my patients said to me, "I'm so alone! I long for acceptance somewhere." Yet the loss of once cherished friends and activities can cause depression and increased isolation.

As with other issues, you need not feel trapped in a group. The choice is yours. You can decide which world you wish to inhabit: the safe one, where you avoid rejection but limit your social and emotional contacts, or the risky one, where you're subject to hurts but experience the full range of life's possibilities. There are always trade-offs. If you choose to return to the "normal" world, you must be prepared to deal with the difficulties you might face. Perhaps you will decide that you want some of both, each being different but sustaining in its own way.

I believe you should use peer groups particularly when you are going through the period of transition and adjustment that occurs with a medical crisis. The group can be extremely valuable until you feel ready to meet the world on your own terms again. It can act as a secure enclosure when you feel fragmented, but you must guard against it becoming a closed circle. The group should facilitate and not hinder your return to "normal" by helping you feel acceptable to yourself, your family, and your friends.

JENNIFER WITHDRAWS FROM THE WORLD

When Jennifer, a twenty-year-old college student with multiple sclerosis, began seeing me, she was closer to complete isolation than she realized. She had quit school, broken up with her boyfriend, set up her own apartment in the basement of her parents' home, and refused phone calls from old friends. She even joined a group at the local chapter of the National Multiple Sclerosis Society and increasingly spent her time with the people she met there. She accomplished all of this within a month of her diagnosis.

Externally, Jennifer had changed very little—she was still a very pretty young woman. But internally, she had relinquished her old self and now moved exclusively with people who she felt would accept her in her new condition. Since she had made these personal changes very quickly, she had barely given herself the opportunity to be rejected. She only anticipated and feared the rejection. In order to be helpful, I needed to understand why Jennifer had moved so hastily.

Once we began to talk, she revealed that inwardly she had always felt "different" from others. (There was no basis in reality for her feelings—they were just part of her personality.) She had always been able to cover her sense of differentness and had created another image for the world. In fact, she used makeup artfully and most people considered her to be beautiful. However, she was afraid that "the truth would come out." She believed she could no longer hide behind her cosmetics. Before, only she knew what she "really" looked like. Now, fearing exposure, she found another way to hide—her support group.

In fact, I became concerned about Jennifer's membership in the group. Rather than being sad, as one might expect, at the changes her illness had caused in her life, she seemed glad. "This group," she told me, "is going to replace my old friends. Now, I'll have real relationships instead of phony ones." On the surface, this seemed wonderful. After all, Jennifer had found a group of friends who were accepting and supportive, who could give her what she needed during this vulnerable period in her life.

But, over the weeks, as she continued to relate how good the group was to her, a theme appeared that worried me. There was one woman in the group, Connie, to whom Jennifer could pour her heart out. Increasingly, Connie became her sole support, to the exclusion of everyone else. "I'm the only one who understands you," Connie told Jennifer repeatedly. "Even your family and friends don't care as much about you as I do."

Jennifer was being seduced. If she continued to believe Connie's statements, she might never see her old friends again. She could even become alienated from the family that she adored.

I knew that Jennifer was fragile—she felt vulnerable and needed acceptance from every quarter. I could not encourage her to distance herself from the group that had filled her needs in time of trouble until she believed she was equally acceptable to her family and old friends.

I began with a question: "What do you think you mean to your old friends besides a heavily made-up face and attractive clothes?"

This opened a discussion of Jennifer's relationships and values. We talked about her former boyfriend and the new man in her life—a fellow MS sufferer who she believed was the one man who could ever accept her. We examined her old and new values, and she discovered that they hadn't changed as much as she had imagined. We reviewed what she had given up as a result of her illness and, finally, what she had been able to hold on to or retrieve.

Slowly but surely, Jennifer began disowning her new image as a "vibrating freak" (her description!) and feeling once again like a whole person. Even with MS, she was still the same individual—and she was a lot better off than she had realized. She didn't have to leave her old world or be forever isolated from it in an attempt to seek a new one.

Jennifer began seeing old friends again, both male and female, testing each relationship by confessing her illness. She drew closer to her mother after several highly emotional talks. She gave up the relationship with the one man who could accept her, realizing that she was perfectly acceptable to a lot of men. While she did not abandon Connie, she did grow to understand why this woman had so zealously attempted to move her away from her "outside" relationships—Connie was lonely and had hoped that Jennifer would fulfill her needs.

Jennifer came by to visit me sporadically, even several years after I had stopped seeing her regularly. Having always felt different, it was difficult for her to accept actually *being* different and being unable to hide it. Yet, she understood her personal dilemma and still made the choice to cope with it in the world at large.

OTHER OPTIONS

How else can you resolve your feelings of isolation? What more can you do to help yourself?

1. Remember, you're never as isolated as you feel. Some friends may drift away but you always have the opportunity and option to make new friends. Also bear in mind that many others feel the way you do. You are not alone in this situation.

2. Think about why others might shy away. Ill people stay away from old friends because they feel vulnerable, less confident, and uncomfortable to have friends see them in distress. Conversely, friends may feel helpless and awkward when faced with your medical condition. You might find it helpful to air your feelings and solicit your friends' perceptions in order to maintain valued old relationships. Let them know how they can include you in their lives.

3. Be realistic. You may not have as much in common with old friends as you once did. If they act uncomfortable around you, you may feel better in their absence. The ability to give others support or tolerate others' discomfort is not universal. You and your family have the opportunity to make new friends who will be valuable to you.

4. Think about how you can reintegrate into society. It's important for you to know where you fit into society now. Consider your situation carefully. Do what is right for you at the moment. Get support from a group, if you need to, but bear in mind that you can alter your position later. Feelings and illnesses are changeable. There is no timetable. You are not locked into any one way of being in the world. You can avoid isolation by reaching out to others, even after you have withdrawn for a period of time.

REMEMBER

- People with chronic illnesses often retreat because it feels safer to do so.
- Withdrawal can lead to isolation.
- Physical isolation can lead to social and emotional isolation.
- Old friends may pull away because they feel distressed and helpless about your condition or they may be uninformed as to how to include you.
- Emotional isolation can cause you to become estranged from familiar habits, dear friendships, and cherished activities.
- Your family may be feeling as isolated as you are.
- Support groups are helpful in alleviating isolation.
- You are never as isolated as you feel.
- You can reach out to others even if you've isolated yourself.

THINGS TO DO

- Prepare yourself for others' ignorance and discomfort.
- Ready a statement to be used at moments when you feel rejected or ignored.
- Let people know how you'd like to be included.

- Join a support group, especially during your adjustment period, but don't let it substitute for your former world. Keep old friends.
- Decide how much support you need and want.
- Be realistic about friends.
- Think about reintegrating into society.

12.

Mastering Your Fear of Death

Death is such a frightening word for all of us. Yet it certainly is no stranger. We have been aware of it all of our lives. We may have confronted it suddenly, swerving to avoid an oncoming truck, or gradually, during the natural course of aging—the first gray hair, the first wrinkle, the first pair of reading glasses. Either way, we probably dismissed the fear of death easily, once we had regained our equilibrium.

With the diagnosis of a long-term illness, however, thoughts of death may be more persistent and frightening. Daily, we are reminded of our vulnerability because of medications or treatments we must take, a lack of mobility, or unremitting pain. What we might have considered a distant eventuality becomes a more plausible and palpable reality.

We may even believe that we have more compelling information now about how and when it will all come about. In one sense, we do know more—the illness could ultimately be fatal. Yet, it may not be. Nevertheless, whether or not the disease is the cause of one's demise, it is now more difficult to tuck away these frightening thoughts for future consideration.

LIVING WITH YOUR FEAR

From the time of the birth of my ill children decades ago, death became like a companion to me. For many years, it hovered somewhere nearby, always looking over my shoulder. I knew it was there, waiting in the wings, but I would not let it stop me or my family from living. We had to face it head-on.

Despite the constant reminders of your physical fragility, you too can live successfully with the fear of death at your side. Many people do it, and do it well. In fact, a relatively new national organization, the National Coalition of Cancer Survivorship, is composed of individuals who never thought they would live as long as they have. Not only are they enjoying fulfilling lives, but they are helping others to do so too.

You'll note that I'm not suggesting you "overcome" or "conquer" the fear—only that you make peace with it. The threat of death can remain a likelihood, even a strong one, yet it does not have to prevent you from delighting in a full and useful life in the time that remains.

Indeed, facing the fear of death can be beneficial to you. It may increase the value of your life; it helps you straighten out your priorities and enhances your appreciation of what you formerly took for granted. When you confront the possibility of dying, you will no longer be frightened to live as fully as you want.

As with all of the issues covered in this book, you have it in your power to take charge of your fear of death. You can be aware of your mortality without letting your fear of it beat you into submission. Even in the face of death, you can remain master of your life. How can you accomplish this difficult task? The first step is to desensitize yourself to the idea of your demise, and the second is to remain in charge of your existence, even in the face of death.

DESENSITIZING YOURSELF

Although many of us have grown up with the belief that "you don't talk about these things," I have found that the more you deal with your death, the less frightening it becomes. The following suggestions may help you desensitize yourself to death.

1. Talk about death. Air your feelings over and over again until the word and topic are no longer upsetting to you. This can occur in peer groups, with a counselor, or carefully among sympathetic family and friends. (Tread gently with loved ones, however, gauging the effect your words are having on them.) Try to use the word—*death*—until it slips off the tongue naturally and dispassionately; until you've drained all the emotion out of it; until it's just a word, like any other.

My wise aunt Bertha repeatedly asked my husband to promise that he be a pallbearer at her funeral. Her request upset us. "Oh, let's not talk about it," we used to say, with a wave of the hand, when she brought up the subject. "It's just too morbid."

But she always replied, with a twinkle and a smile, "Talking about it isn't going to make it happen any sooner!" And she was right.

2. Help others who are very sick. In assisting those who are more desperately ill than you, you can overcome your squeamishness around death. You can see that it's possible to die with dignity and integrity.

When I decided to work with people struggling with the most severe medical problems, I knew I couldn't be afraid to discuss death with them. This was what they wanted to talk about. Because of my experiences, I was desensitized. Talking about death didn't frighten me.

3. Write about it. Writing is a powerful form of self-expression, one that may be even more valuable than talking. When you write, you literally take the thought out of your mind and put it somewhere else. Writing helps you organize unmanageable events and feelings and reduces physical and mental stress. Of course, it cannot provide you with the emotional support you might receive from another, but it can certainly help you become familiar and comfortable with your fear.

As I mentioned in chapter 5, my daughter, Linda, wrote about her fears in the months preceding her final heart surgery. After her death, I found a notebook overflowing with her thoughts about the possibility of death. Her final entry, the poem I shared, expressed her fears and hopes, yet it was not filled with apprehension. It was Linda's way of preparing herself for any outcome. She went into the operating room with a smile; the possibility of death had not stopped her from living.

4. Plan for it. You can plan for your death and still enjoy your life. This strategy has been extremely helpful for many of my patients. They were actually planning for life—theirs and their loved ones'.

Some wanted to decide how their funerals would take place. They chose caskets and headstones in advance or wrote letters to their families that were to be read during the service. Others arranged for their children's futures; they helped select the schools they would attend. Still others divided their precious and sentimental possessions in anticipation of their deaths and made sure their wills were in order. Peace of mind comes with feeling one has completed any unfinished business.

TAKING CHARGE

When you talk about the fear of death, what are you really afraid of? In all of my years of practice, I have observed that people actually fear two eventualities more than death itself:

1. *The end of living:* Being unable to complete one's life's plans.
2. *The process of dying:* The possibility of coping with pain or increased debilitation.

Some people cannot bear the thought of a life filled with pain or severe physical disability. To them, it is the ultimate loss of control. Yet, if they can recapture some of their former power, they discover that life, as difficult as it may have become, is worth the battle. They take control of their lives, in the face of overwhelming odds, wresting it away from the ever increasing possibility of death. They may be dying, but in the meantime they're living as fully as they can.

Most likely, it's not so much the fear of death as it is how you will handle the rest of your life that scares you so. Once you regain control, you will realize that you no longer fear death because you have learned to manage your life. You may find the following suggestions helpful:

1. Plan for the future. Even though you may see death on the horizon, daily events and outings (to the movies, to dinner, to your child's school) still require planning and provide impetus for living. Long-range planning, as mentioned above, can also be helpful. The realization that eventually you will be separated from your loved ones can motivate you to use your time more purposefully. Life goes on as long as possible.

2. *Talk about what you will miss.* Paradoxical as it may seem, grieving losses can be healing. Many of my patients have been able to talk about what they would miss if they died: a daughter's college graduation, watching grandchildren grow. They angrily express how their illness has fouled up their plans and foreshortened their futures.

Yet, interestingly enough, they lament their fates while carefully planning for next month's Christmas dinner or choosing tomorrow night's movie. These individuals realize that even if they do experience fear and loss, life still moves along. The anticipation of death does not preclude living in the moment. They are not mutually exclusive.

3. *Maintain your dignity and integrity.* It is difficult to remain in charge of your life, but you are the only one who will decide how you're to live. Even under the worst of circumstances, knowing that the final choices are up to you will help you maintain your dignity and integrity. When you take responsibility for decisions affecting your health, you remain in control. You will remain true to yourself.

4. *Face death as you have faced life.* This is not the time to try a "better" way of coping or to live up to others' expectations. That only increases tension. You must do and say what is familiar, what feels right to you—not what will please others. And you must not feel a failure if you have disappointed others. This is your life, after all.

When Dolores, one of my dearest and closest friends, was dying of lung cancer a few years ago, she asked me if it was all right for her to stop doing creative imagery, a relaxation

technique that cancer patients often use. She had been try-
ing to please her psychiatrist, but felt extremely uncom-
fortable with this practice. The concept was totally alien to
Dolores's concrete, realistic way of relating to the world.
Because it was so unfamiliar, it was not relaxing her at all.
In fact, it made her more tense than before.

In going along with someone else's idea about how to
relax, Dolores had unwittingly forfeited some of her own
integrity—something that had been a vital part of her being.
I urged her to do whatever felt comfortable for her.

5. *Confront your fears in your own way.* When in dire
circumstances, it's common for people to search for anything that will help them—the "perfect" solution. In truth,
no single solution exists. There are as many ways of reacting to the fear of death as there are people on the earth.

Still, struggling to cope with your own suffering, you
may look with envy at others who seem to be managing
more successfully. You may wonder if they have some hidden secret or the right answer. Well, the truth is, the answer
is not hidden at all. And it's not a secret either. Simply confront your fears in your own way. If, as I explained on p. 26,
avoiding feels better, then that's the way you must cope. If
you're in a confronting frame of mind, then bring your feelings out in the open. Staying true to your coping style, even
in face of death, will help you maintain your integrity.

6. *Become aware of symbolic expressions.* You may be
expressing your fears without being fully aware of it. Seemingly innocuous phrases—such as "I was hoping to be at
Mary Jane's wedding" or "I had been looking forward to taking a cruise in my old age"—are coded ways of verbalizing
your fear of death. Everyone knows, without your disclosing it directly, what you are thinking. When you use such
symbolic language, you are not hiding or suppressing your
fears. You are letting them out.

Dreams are another symbolic way to manifest your feelings. While in a dream-state, your mind helps you to confront your fears. As the unconscious takes over, you may find yourself coping with issues you could never bring yourself to speak out loud. Whereas you may believe that you have tucked away these thoughts in the deep recesses of your mind, your dreams may push them into the foreground. This can be good. Your unconscious is acting like a safety valve, helping you work out your worst fears symbolically.

On the other hand, some people cannot use enough words to express their fears of death. Rose literally talked nonstop in my office. When she was home, she continued her outpouring to anyone who would listen. She didn't need dreams to help her work out her issues symbolically. She did it day and night on her own; she held nothing back. Understanding that this was Rose's way of working through her fears, neither her family nor I stopped her.

7. Temper your expectations of science. Because of high expectations of medical technology in our society, it is particularly difficult to accept the inevitability of death. We truly believe that when we become ill there must be a superdrug or exotic surgical procedure that will save us. Or we believe that, if we can only just stay alive long enough, someone will come up with a cure that doesn't presently exist.

Of course, rationally, we all expect to die someday. But do we also, irrationally, believe that we will be "saved" forever? I'm afraid the answer to that question is a resounding yes. Our illogical hopes are based on amazing scientific advances that have produced great results in the last few years. Many miraculous medical and surgical procedures are available today that didn't exist a decade or two ago. Heart, liver, kidney, lung, and other organ transplants are now feasible. Drugs like interferon can halt certain types of cancer. Gene therapy holds much promise for the future.

Still, we must be careful in our expectations. We should recognize realistically that these procedures are life-extenders, not cures in the traditional sense. And they are not appropriate for everyone.

8. *Accept the idea of remission rather than "cure."* New medical procedures either bypass a diseased organ or correct or replace an old one. Powerful drugs can attack an illness in such a way that you may appear "disease free" for years. Scientific advances can extend your life, even to the normal life span, but you must be careful to recognize that you are not "cured"—instead, you are in remission.

If you do believe that you are cured and your disease eventually returns, you may be deeply shocked and disappointed. I have seen many patients experience this pain unnecessarily. Rather, I encourage my patients who feel "well" to accept that they are not cured but in remission. This holds out the possibility that the illness might return, even though you hope it won't.

Accepting remission is beneficial in two other ways. First, it helps you to take better care of your health—you know that you must remain vigilant. You may not prevent the return of the disease, but you may be able to slow its progression. Besides, you'll feel as good as possible. Second, when you believe that you are in remission, you can plan your life more realistically. If you accept the possibility that the disease may visit again, and if it does, you will be better prepared to cope with it.

Remission can be almost as good as a cure. It can even last up to forty or fifty years. I have seen this many times. The medical or surgical treatment has, in the words of many physicians, bought you time—sometimes a lifetime's worth.

9. Never give up the prerogative to make decisions, despite a desire to let them go. To maintain control of your life, even under the most dire circumstances, never give up your right to make decisions. You must hold on to this prerogative with all of your might, for there may be times when you feel like letting go and allowing someone else to take over. As long as you maintain your ability to make decisions, you will stay in charge of your life. If you give it up, you are in a sense giving up on living—something I'm sure you don't want to do.

10. Ask the hard questions. If you must make a medical decision that requires you to calculate the quality of your life, then ask yourself the hard questions. Try to discover what lies ahead: How risky is the treatment? What will your life be like if you take it? What if you don't? Do the benefits outweigh the financial, physical, and emotional risks? Can you balance the two?

If a decision is too difficult to make entirely on your own or even with your family, seek input from someone who is emotionally uninvolved—a physician or counselor. It may stir up anxiety to receive some answers you may not want to hear, but in the long run, when you're apprised of the truth, you will be better prepared to face what lies ahead. Remember, even if you ask for advice, you are still in charge of what you do with it.

11. Stay close to loved ones. It is often normal for someone who is dying to distance himself from loved ones. It's a way of lessening the pain of separation. One of my patients with advanced breast cancer took this approach with her young daughter. "Maybe Evelyn will miss me less this way," she said.

When you push others away, you all lose the opportunity to experience closeness and intimacy. Although you may believe that you are sparing your family pain, they may not understand your sudden coolness. This can hurt them more, especially if they feel they are losing you. Use this rare moment to be good to yourself and your loved ones. Express your love.

12. Look for elements of hope. Even in the face of death, your task is to survive with hope. Hope increases the quality of life, no matter how long you have to live. I have found that most of my patients who faced death spoke frequently of life. They talked about their children and spouses. They worried about their appearance and their futures. They wondered if they still had time to take long postponed trips. They continued to seek solutions to longtime family problems. In the face of death, they were embracing life and holding fast.

Besides, if there's a 5 percent survival rate for a disease, there's no reason to believe that you are not among that 5 percent. Hope fuels the will to live, which may have a positive effect on the course of your illness.

13. Leave room for miracles. It is possible for miracles to occur. Many people live well beyond their prognoses; told that they might be dead within a few months, they delight years later in laughing at these dire predictions. Sometimes these reprieves occur because of misdiagnosis; sometimes they're the result of outstanding treatment; sometimes they're due to life-style changes; sometimes they just happen.

Tom, the young lupus patient I wrote about in chapter 5, was given six months to live—eleven years ago! He clearly went into remission and extended his life. He knows he's not cured, but that hasn't stopped him from leading a full and happy life. Perhaps his brush with death provided him with an additional incentive to experience life to the fullest.

14. Arrange to die at home, if possible. Dying at home, surrounded by the one's closest and dearest, has benefits for all. Rather than being isolated in a sterile environment with strangers, at home you can be in comfortable, familiar surroundings with people who love and care about you more than any professional can. This arrangement is even better for your family. Members can spend time with you and talk to you at will.

Companies such as Quantum (in twenty-two cities nationwide) provide sophisticated medical support at home, should you require it. There are also excellent home-nursing services available to help you and your family in your final days.

FRANCES CHOOSES LIFE

Frances hung on to her decision-making prerogative for dear life. It carried her through what could have been her darkest days. Maintaining her integrity in face of death gave her the physical and mental stamina she required to face a second kidney transplant and whatever followed.

Frances first came into my office ranting, raging, and raving. All I could make out initially was her distress about her "overprotective" husband and children.

"They don't care about my feelings at all," she exclaimed. "All they care about is themselves. Don't they realize what they're asking me to do? Don't they know that I'm not up to all those horrible procedures again? I'm definitely never having another kidney transplant again, and there's nothing they can do or say that will make me change my mind. Not even Ron sending me here to see you is going to make a difference."

"But if your mind is already made up," I asked, "what are you doing in my office?"

"I only came to please my husband. He begged me to come, but it's going to make absolutely no difference, period! I'm not undergoing a second transplant."

I asked Frances about her previous surgery and she explained that she had almost died several years ago, during the first transplant. "But now that kidney isn't working anymore," she said, "and dialysis isn't effective either. My choices are to risk the dangers and pain of a second transplant or not have it and die."

To complicate matters, her first grandchild was about to be born. This was the issue that really brought Frances in to see me. "More than anything else," she told me, "I want to hold that baby."

It was easy for me to discern that Frances had a strong personality, which I would help her use at this critical time in her life. I also realized that rather than helping her make her own decisions—so vital to her well-being—her family was trying to make them for her. She became angry and intransigent because they were wresting from her control over her life. She found this loss even more intolerable than facing surgery or even dying. If I could help her regain control, she would be in charge again and would be able to make the decision she wanted. More than anything else, she needed to be at peace with the decision.

I said, "Frances, I feel I need to remind you that actually, no matter what the doctors or your family try to persuade you to do, the final decision to undergo this operation is yours. They might argue their point of view compellingly, but really this decision is in your hands and no one can take it away from you."

As the truth of my statement sank in, Frances calmed visibly. When she left my office, rather than being overwrought, she seemed quiet and pensive. I looked forward to seeing her the following week.

During our next meeting, it was clear that Frances's extreme agitation had subsided. She spoke in an organized manner, clearly and firmly. Before she said it, intuitively I knew that she had reached a decision.

"All week I thought about what we had discussed," she explained. "I thought it over alone, without talking to Ron or my children. I've made up my mind. I'm going to have the surgery."

I was rather surprised, given Frances's adamant statement of the previous week. "Are you sure?" I asked.

"Yes, quite sure. I decided to do whatever will give me the best chance of holding my grandchild. Everything else is predicated on that.

"The baby is like a catalyst for me. If I can't see my grandchild, if I die before he's born, I want to leave him my legacy, something the child will remember me by. This week, I decided that I don't want him to remember me as a coward or a weakling. I can't bear that thought. If I don't try the surgery and take my only opportunity for life, no matter what the pain, it would be a cowardly act, like committing suicide. The legacy I want to leave is that no matter what, one chooses life."

Having made this decision, Frances had to set the date of her surgery, although there was only about a month's leeway. Her daughter was due to deliver within weeks. But, perhaps more crucial, the operation had to be performed as soon as a kidney became available. Frances was hoping that her grandchild would arrive before the kidney, because, realistically, her odds for survival were slim. (This was a few years ago, when repeat transplants were highly risky procedures.)

This could have been an agonizing period for Frances and her family, but it wasn't. Once she had decided on her own (and she made that point very clear to me), she and her family awaited the surgery peacefully.

Frances and I used our time together to help her understand why her family had pressed her so hard and why she had reacted so vehemently. Although they never told her directly, their coerciveness was their way of showing her how much they loved her. They had hoped, in so doing, to give her strength to undergo the difficult procedure.

For her part, Frances needed to recognize that, although she loved them very much and would do anything to please them, her need to maintain control and integrity—especially at this stage in her life—superseded all else. This sense of herself would give her strength to undergo what she had feared so much. Having needed a powerful reason to live, she found one in the maintenance of her integrity.

Frances spent the next few weeks quite relaxed. As she went into the hospital to be readied for surgery, her grandchild was born. She was thrilled and spent several happy hours on the phone with her daughter. Unfortunately, she never had the opportunity to know if the surgery would work. She died the next day, while awaiting the arrival of her new kidney.

Despite its sad ending, I found Frances's story uplifting. Even in the face of death, she had maintained control over her life. What was ultimately most important to her was not how she died, but how she lived. She would not give up being herself until the end. Having taken control of her life and made her own decision, she could face anything—even death—with dignity.

Learning to live with the fear of death is probably the hardest task we can accomplish in our lives. When we no longer fear it, we are free to live the rest of our lives as fully as we wish. In coping with long-term illness, I believe that is all we can ask.

REMEMBER

- Death is frightening to all of us but becomes even more threatening when you are diagnosed with a long-term illness.

- It is possible to live happily while confronting your fear of death.
- The fear can even be beneficial, helping you to set priorities.
- People fear the end of living and the process of dying more than they do death itself.

THINGS TO DO

- Desensitize yourself to death.
  - Talk about it.
  - Help others.
  - Write about it.
  - Plan for it.
- Take charge of your fear by taking control of your life.
  - Plan for the future.
  - Talk about what you'll miss.
  - Maintain your dignity and integrity.
  - Face death as you have faced life.
  - Confront your fears in your own way.
  - Become aware of symbolic expressions.
  - Temper your expectations of science.
  - Accept the idea of remission.
  - Never give up your prerogative to make decisions.
  - Ask the hard questions.
  - Stay close to loved ones.
  - Look for elements of hope.
  - Leave room for miracles.
  - Arrange to die at home, if possible.
  - Live life to the fullest.

Epilogue:
A Message of Hope

As we began this book, I asked you to pretend that you were seated in a chair, facing me, and that we were engaged in conversation. In finishing, I now feel that we have brought our relationship full circle. It is as if you have been my client and are now terminating your work with me. And, just as in the final session of a therapeutic relationship, I would like to sum up what we have accomplished together and to take this opportunity to add some final words of wisdom.

In a therapeutic partnership, each of us has a role to play. Mine was to help you discover insights into your problems at this time of trouble; yours was to think about yourself in new ways. I must give credit where it's due: your part was harder than mine.

I hope that I have helped you to understand what you are experiencing and how you are reacting as a result of your illness. This of course doesn't mean that your problems are over—only that you can focus on them more clearly and perhaps find better ways to deal with them.

Each of us resolves challenges in our own way, at our own pace, and on our own terms. I hope you have learned how *you* cope, and, given your circumstances, I hope you appreciate that you are not doing so badly after all. Reading about how others have faced similar dilemmas doesn't mean their way is better and therefore should be emulated. Instead, I have presented these examples to encourage you to develop your own solutions to your unique problems.

In truth, even when you feel everything you're doing is wrong, you are actually experiencing your struggle. This is what each of us does as we face the enormous challenges that long-term illness has set before us. This is what each of us does as we grapple with maintaining integrity and control over our lives in these difficult circumstances.

If I am really saying good-bye, what do I want you to take away from our time together? Here are a few thoughts I hope you will always remember:

- It is always frightening to face the unknown, but perhaps now, armed with new information and some workable strategies, it will be less so.
- You did not seek this disease; it was handed to you. Your mind is naturally resisting the physical, psychological, and practical changes it has forced upon you. Recognizing your resistance can help you overcome it and get on with your life.
- Even though it may be your strongest wish, your problems will not disappear overnight. You are in the midst of a dynamic and difficult process, and your primary goal is to get through it.
- If you are in crisis, guard against making drastic decisions now that will affect the rest of your life. Your

medical condition may not be as bad as you anticipate. It could even be a lot better!

- You can be helpful to your family by understanding their limits and showing your appreciation for their efforts.
- Your relationship with your doctor and her staff should be one of mutual respect and cooperation. But you must always remain in charge of medical decisions.
- You can regain a sense of control over your life as soon as you set reachable and realistic goals. Even getting through the next hour may be such a goal.
- You can attain a new (and satisfying) identity, but first you must let go of the old one.
- If you find ways to be valuable to your family and the community, you will never become a burden.
- Society will not reject you unless you reject yourself. You can live comfortably with a long-term disease as long as you always consider yourself a person of value to yourself, your family, and society.
- Your family wishes to get rid of the situation caused by your illness, not you.
- Depression is anger turned inward. If it goes unrecognized and unexpressed, it can be insidious, draining whatever energy you have. Releasing that anger should also release your energy potential.
- You can choose isolation from your family and old friends, but you can also choose to remain in the mainstream. It is not easy, but it is up to you to show others how to accept you.
- Living with a chronic illness can be more frightening than dying. But as long as you are alive, you have the opportunity to meet the challenges of living.
- If you have reflected on the eight fears represented here, you will have confronted most of what is over-

whelming and terrifying for you. This should result in your feeling less anxious and more in control.

By now, you should know a lot more about yourself and your situation. I hope you're feeling that you can and will take charge of your life. Rather than being a slave to your fears, I hope I have helped you to master them. You have it in your power to do so; the choice is yours.

References

American Heart Association. 1994. *AHA Family Guide to Stroke.* New York: Times.

Cousins, N. 1979. *Anatomy of an Illness as Perceived by the Patient: Reflections on Healing and Regeneration.* New York: Norton.

Fawzy, F.I., N. Cousins, N.W. Fawzy et al. 1990(a). A structured psychiatric intervention for cancer patients. I. Changes over time in methods of coping and affective disturbance. *Archives of General Psychiatry* 47:720–25.

Fawzy, F.I., M.E. Kemeny, N.W. Fawzy et al. 1990(b). A structured psychiatric intervention for cancer patients. II. Changes over time in immunological measures. *Archives of General Psychiatry* 47:729–35.

Goffman, E. 1974. *Stigma: Notes on the Management of a Spoiled Identity.* New York: Aronson.

Goleman, D. December 24, 1991. Hope emerges as key to success in life. *The New York Times*, p. C1.

Goleman, D. December 15, 1992. New light on how stress erodes health. *The New York Times*, p. C1.

Hill, D.R., K. Kelleher, and S.A. Shumaker. 1992. Psychosocial interventions in adult patients with coronary heart disease and cancer: A literature review. *General Hospital Psychiatry* 14(6S):28S–42S.

Jellinek, M., M.D. Trill, S. Passik et al. 1992. The need for multidisciplinary training in counseling the mentally ill: Report of the Training Committee of the Linda Pollin Foundation. *General Hospital Psychiatry* 14(6S):3S–10S.

Koocher, G.P. 1980. Pediatric cancer: Psychosocial problems and the high cost of helping. *Journal of Clinical Child Psychology* 9:2–5.

Lansky, S.B., et al. 1978. Childhood cancer: Parental discord and divorce. *Pediatrics* 62:184–88.

Levenson, J.L. 1992. Psychosocial interventions in chronic medical illness: An overview of outcome research. *General Hospital Psychiatry* 14(6S):43S–49S.

Minuchin, S. 1974. *Family Therapy Techniques.* Cambridge, MA: Harvard University Press.

National Center for Health Statistics. 1990. *Vital and Health Statistics. Current Estimates from the National Health Interview Survey, 1989.* Series 10, No. 176, U.S. Department of Health and Human Services, DHHS Pub. No. (PHS) 90-1504, Hyattsville, MD.

National Institute of Mental Health and the Linda Pollin Foundation. Proceedings, June 21–23, 1989. *Counseling the Chronic Medically Ill: Needs, Barriers, Strategies for the Future,* Chevy Chase, MD.

National Institute of Mental Health and the Linda Pollin Foundation. Proceedings from the Second Annual Workshop, June 17–19, 1990. *Model Curriculum in Medical Crisis Counseling,* Chevy Chase, MD.

National Institute of Mental Health and the Linda Pollin Foundation. Proceedings from the Third Annual Workshop, June 25–26, 1991. *Health Policy and Medical Crisis Counseling,* Chevy Chase, MD.

Pollin, I. 1984. Community-based social work with the chronically ill. In Richard J. Estes, ed., *Health Care and the Social Services: Social Work Practice in Health Care.* St. Louis: Warren H. Green.

Pollin, I., et al. 1992. Model curriculum in Medical Crisis Counseling. *General Hospital Psychiatry* 14(6S):11S–27S.

Pollin, I., and J. Holland. 1992. A model for counseling the medically ill: The Linda Pollin Foundation approach. *General Hospital Psychiatry* 14(6S):1S–2S.

Rosenbaum, E.H. 1982. *Living with Cancer.* New York: New American Library.

Rosenberg, G. 1989. The future of Medical Crisis Counseling: Services for the chronically ill, their families, and significant others. *Linda Pollin Memorial Lecture,* University of Maryland at Baltimore, School of Social Work.

Spiegel, D., J.R. Bloom, H.C. Kramer, and E. Gottheil. 1989. Effects of psychosocial treatment on survival of patients with metastatic breast cancer. *The Lancet* 2:888–91.

Strain, J.J. 1993. Psychotherapy and medical conditions. In D. Goleman and J. Gurin, eds., *Mind Body Medicine: How to Use Your Mind for Better Health.* Yonkers, NY: Consumer Reports Books, pp. 368–83.

Tavris, C. 1989. *Anger: The Misunderstood Emotion,* rev. ed. New York: Simon & Schuster.

Worden, J.W., and A.D. Weisman. 1984. Preventive psychosocial intervention with newly diagnosed cancer patients. *General Hospital Psychiatry* 6:243–49.

Index

Self-image: and being a "sick" person, 115–24; components of,
113; consequences of loss of,
114–15; and family/caregiver
relationships, 37, 41, 125–26;
and fears of chronic illness, 11,
12–13; forging a new, 117, 122–
24, 251; and grief, 117–20; and
letting go of your old identity,
117, 120–22, 251; and losses you
may face, 118–20; and making a
new life, 126–31; mastering
fears of loss of, 113–32; stages in
adopting a new, realistic,
116–24; and stigma, 12–13, 159,
251; and support groups, 121
Specialists, 59–67
Spiegel, David, 10, 88
Stigma: and anger, 161; buying
into the, 160; effects of, 158–60;
and family/caregiver relationships, 37, 160, 161, 169; and
fears of chronic illness, 12–13;
and guilt, 162, 167; and isolation, 160–62, 219; and legal
action, 172; mastering fears of,
158–78; and self-image, 12–13,
159, 251; and stress, 161; and
support groups, 168; and taking
charge, 163–77; and victimization, 160
Stress: and anger, 25–26; and control, 94, 99–100, 112; and coping
style, 26–30, 33; identifying, 94,
99–100, 112; reduction of, 94,
102–5, 112; and stigma, 161
Support/support groups: and
anger, 208–9, 212; benefits of,

224–25; and control, 94, 108–9,
112; and coping style, 30; and
dealing with fears/feelings, 10,
14; and dependency, 146; and
the doctor-patient partnership,
62; and family/caregiver relationships, 38, 42, 46, 47, 53, 55,
209, 212; and goals, 226; and
home nursing services, 244; and
isolation, 14, 223–27; and leaving the group, 226–27; and medical improvements, 10; and the
process for coping, 30; purpose
of, 227; and self–image, 121;
sources of, 226; and stigma, 168
Surgery, 71
Symbolic expressions, 239–40

Taking stock. *See* Assessment
Tavris, Carol, 13
Tension. *See* Anger; Stress
Things to do: and abandonment,
197; and anger, 217; and control,
112; and death, 248; and dependency, 157; and the doctor-
patient partnership, 81; and
family/caregiver relationships,
57; and isolation/withdrawal,
231–32; and self-image, 132; and
stigma, 177–78
Tranquilizers, 104–5, 200, 206
Treatment, 60, 68–69, 88, 137

Victimization, 73–74, 160, 202,
212

Withdrawal. *See* Depression;
Isolation